# Extrapolating Evidence of
# HEALTH
## Information Technology
## Savings and Costs

Federico Girosi

Robin Meili

Richard Scoville

Sponsored by Cerner Corporation, General Electric, Hewlett-Packard, Johnson & Johnson, and Xerox

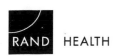

RAND HEALTH

The research described in this report was conducted within RAND Health and sponsored by a consortium of private companies, including Cerner Corporation, General Electric, Hewlett-Packard, Johnson & Johnson, and Xerox.

**Library of Congress Cataloging-in-Publication Data**

Girosi, Federico.
    Extrapolating evidence of health information technology savings and costs /
Federico Girosi, Robin Meili, Richard Scoville.
        p. cm.
    "MG-410."
    Includes bibliographical references.
    ISBN 0-8330-3851-6 (pbk. : alk. paper)
    1. Medical records—Data processing.  I. Meili, Robin. II. Scoville, Richard P.
III.Title.
        [DNLM: 1. Medical Records Systems, Computerized—economics—United States.
    2. Cost-Benefit Analysis—United States.  WX 173 G527e 2005]

R864.G57 2005
651.5'04261—dc22

                                                                                2005024409

The RAND Corporation is a nonprofit research organization providing objective analysis and effective solutions that address the challenges facing the public and private sectors around the world. RAND's publications do not necessarily reflect the opinions of its research clients and sponsors.

**RAND®** is a registered trademark.

A profile of RAND Health, abstracts of its publications, and ordering information can be found on the RAND Health home page at www.rand.org/health.

Published 2005 by the RAND Corporation
1776 Main Street, P.O. Box 2138, Santa Monica, CA 90407-2138
1200 South Hayes Street, Arlington, VA 22202-5050
201 North Craig Street, Suite 202, Pittsburgh, PA 15213-1516
RAND URL: http://www.rand.org/
To order RAND documents or to obtain additional information, contact
Distribution Services: Telephone: (310) 451-7002;
Fax: (310) 451-6915; Email: order@rand.org

# Preface

It is widely believed that broad adoption of Electronic Medical Record Systems (EMR-S) will lead to significant healthcare savings, reduce medical errors, and improve health, effectively transforming the U.S. healthcare system. Yet, adoption of EMR-S has been slow and appears to lag the effective application of information technology (IT) and related transformations seen in other industries, such as banking, retail, and telecommunications. In 2003, RAND Health began a broad study to better understand the role and importance of EMR-S in improving health and reducing healthcare costs, and to help inform government actions that could maximize EMR-S benefits and increase its use.

This monograph provides the technical details and results of one component of that study. In it, we quantify national-level efficiency savings (what results from the ability to perform the same task with fewer resources [money, time, personnel, etc.]) brought about by using Health Information Technology (HIT) and compare them to the costs the nation has to incur in order to be able to realize those savings. Related documents are as follows:

- Richard Hillestad, James Bigelow, Anthony Bower, Federico Girosi, Robin Meili, Richard Scoville, and Roger Taylor, "Can Electronic Medical Record Systems Transform Healthcare? Potential Health Benefits, Savings, and Costs," *Health Affairs,* Vol. 24, No. 5, September 14, 2005.
- Roger Taylor, Anthony Bower, Federico Girosi, James Bigelow, Kateryna Fonkych, and Richard Hillestad, "Promoting Health Information Technology: Is There a Case for More-Aggressive Government Action?" *Health Affairs,* Vol. 24, No. 5, September 14, 2005.
- James Bigelow et al., "Technical Executive Summary in Support of 'Can Electronic Medical Record Systems Transform Healthcare?' and 'Promoting Health Information Technology'," *Health Affairs,* Web Exclusive, September 14, 2005.
- James Bigelow, Kateryna Fonkych, Constance Fung, and Jason Wang, *Analysis of Healthcare Interventions That Change Patient Trajectories,* Santa Monica, Calif.: RAND Corporation, MG-408-HLTH, 2005.

- Kateryna Fonkych and Roger Taylor, *The State and Pattern of Health Information Technology Adoption,* Santa Monica, Calif.: RAND Corporation, MG-409-HLTH, 2005.
- Richard Scoville, Roger Taylor, Robin Meili, and Richard Hillestad, *How HIT Can Help: Process Change and the Benefits of Healthcare Information Technology,* Santa Monica, Calif.: RAND Corporation, TR-270-HLTH, 2005.
- Anthony G. Bower, *The Diffusion and Value of Healthcare Information Technology,* Santa Monica, Calif.: RAND Corporation, MG-272-HLTH, 2005.

The monograph should be of interest to healthcare IT professionals, other healthcare executives and researchers, and officials in the government responsible for health policy.

This research was sponsored by a generous consortium of private companies: Cerner Corporation, General Electric, Hewlett-Packard, Johnson & Johnson, and Xerox. A steering group headed by Dr. David Lawrence, a retired CEO of Kaiser Permanente, provided review and guidance throughout the project. The right to publish any results was retained by the RAND Corporation. This research was conducted by RAND Health, a division of the RAND Corporation. A profile of RAND Health, abstracts of its publications, and ordering information can be found at www.rand.org/health.

# Contents

# Figures

# Tables

# Summary

Health Information Technology[1] (HIT) is receiving a great deal of attention, and many would like to see it play an expanded role in providing care. The result of our effort to gain a better understanding of the potential of HIT to transform the provision of healthcare is documented in Hillestad et al. (2005), and the policy implications of that work are reported in Taylor et al. (2005). In this monograph, we expand on some of the quantitative aspects of the Hillestad et al. and Taylor et al. research, providing detailed supporting material on the following four related aspects of that research:

- **Extrapolation of savings to the national level and projection of savings into the future (Chapter Two):** The research in Hillestad et al. (2005) focuses on the benefits and costs that would accrue to and be sustained by the nation as a whole as a result of widespread adoption of HIT. Our first step is to provide a methodological framework to scale empirical evidence on the effect of HIT at the national level and to project it into the future. A key element of this framework is a projection for the rates of adoption of HIT in the inpatient setting and in the ambulatory/outpatient setting. This component is developed using models of HIT adoption and analysis of historical data found in Bower (2005) and Fonkych and Taylor (2005), and in work developed by Hillestad, Taylor, and others as part of the same project. Projections of HIT adoption can then be combined with data on specific effects of HIT at the provider level and on national expenditures to provide projections of future national savings in certain health sectors. An important lesson that emerges from this chapter is that realistic estimates of savings must take into account the relatively slow diffusion of HIT: Although large savings may accrue once adoption is almost complete, the

---

[1] We use Health Information Technology (HIT) and Electronic Medical Record System (EMR-S) interchangeably in this report. An EMR-S, as we use it here, includes the Electronic Medical Record (EMR), containing current and historical patient information; Clinical Decision Support (CDS), which provides reminders and best-practice guidance for treatment; and a Central Data Repository, which stores the EMR information. It also includes information technology–enabled functions such as Computerized Physician Order Entry (CPOE), which facilitates orders tied to patient-information and -treatment pathways.

average yearly savings accruing between now and that time are smaller, usually 50 percent smaller.

Clearly, the methodology developed in this chapter is useless without a set of empirical findings. Therefore, we also document in this chapter the extensive literature search we performed, seeking evidence on the effects of HIT at the provider level. An important conclusion from this section is that much of the available evidence is incomplete and cannot be scaled to the national level because key measures are lacking: Out of more than 1,400 screened articles, we were able to extract only 42 findings that could be used as input to our model of national savings.

- **Benefits of HIT (Chapter Three)**: The benefits we focus on in this document are efficiency savings that are enabled by HIT, whereas the HIT-related benefits discussed in Bigelow et al. (2005b) are in health improvement. In this context, *efficiency savings* are what results from the ability to perform the same task with fewer resources (money, time, personnel, etc.). From the evidence found in the literature search, we consider savings from 10 different sources: five for the inpatient sector (such as savings coming from reduction in length of stay or increases in nurse productivity) and five for the outpatient/ambulatory sector (such as reduction in transcription costs or drug expenditures). For each of these sources, we detail the nature of the data and the extrapolation procedure and report the *potential savings*—that is, the savings that would accrue if the HIT adoption rate were to jump to 100 percent overnight—as well as the mean yearly savings over the next 15 years. When we sum the savings over the 10 sources, we find a potential savings of about $80 billion, with a mean yearly savings of about $40 billion. Three-fourths of the savings are found in the inpatient sector, coming mostly from reductions in length of stay and increases in nurses' productivity. While these numbers are fairly large when compared with the cost of HIT adoption, documented in Chapter Four, we note that most of the effects of HIT are not very large: Typical reductions in expenditures are 10 to 15 percent, showing that the reason for the large savings lies in the large national expenditures, rather than in large HIT effects.

- **Costs of HIT (Chapter Four)**: The efficiency savings documented in Chapter Three need to be compared with the costs the nation has to incur in order to be able to realize those savings. We estimated these costs using a modeling framework analogous to the one developed for the extrapolation of savings. Our cost data were gathered through the literature or given to us by providers. For the inpatient sector, the data suggest that, in order to acquire an EMR-S, a hospital might spend between 1.8 and 3 percent of its yearly operating expenditures for an average period of four years. This puts the projected cumulative national expenditures on inpatient EMR-S between now and 15 years from now at $97.4 billion, with a mean yearly cost of $6.5 billion. By comparison, costs in the outpatient/ambulatory sector are much lower, by a factor of almost one-sixth. The average cost per physician of an ambulatory EMR-S estimated from our data is about $22,000, which implies a cumulative cost over the next 15 years of $17.2 billion and a mean yearly cost of $1.1 billion.

- **Incentives for Adoption of HIT (Chapter Five):** Even a cursory look at benefits and costs shows that the savings enabled by widespread HIT adoption are significantly larger than the expenditures on EMR-S that would have to be incurred in order for those savings to materialize. If we aggregate over all healthcare sectors, we project mean annual savings of almost $42 billion, while mean annual costs are about $7.6 billion. Obviously, these numbers would be larger if the adoption of HIT happened at a faster rate than is projected. Therefore, we studied what might be the effect of those financial incentives presented to providers that lower the cost of EMR-S and quicken the pace of HIT adoption. In particular, we considered per-encounter payments to physicians who adopt an EMR-S and percentage subsidies to hospitals. The estimation of costs and benefits of such incentives is particularly difficult, because it requires knowledge of how sensitive providers are to the price of EMR-S, something that has never been measured. Despite this uncertainty, relying on sensitivity analysis we conclude that, even under pessimistic assumptions, programs aimed at incentivizing HIT adoption can deliver benefits that outweigh costs. A general result that does not depend on the size of the behavioral response of physicians is that incentive programs are more likely to be cost-effective if they start early and do not last long, but are sizable. This result is intuitive and depends on the "contagious" nature of technology adoption: The number of new adopters is proportional to the number of current adopters. Therefore, a spike in adoption in one year has long-lasting effects, which propagate well into the future. This implies that, even if an incentive program lasts only one year, if it is sizable enough to produce a spike in adoption, it will lead to benefits that will accumulate over many years to follow, while the cost is incurred in one year only.

The chapters outlined above are followed by a summary chapter. Readers who are interested in the policy issues related to HIT adoption and/or who want to put this document in a more general perspective are encouraged to read Hillestad et al. (2005) and Taylor et al. (2005).

Throughout this document, we refer to a number of Excel spreadsheets that contain additional information and may allow the user to interact with some of our models. The spreadsheets are part of the online version of the monograph at http://www.rand.org/publications/MG/MG410 and are cited by their file names.

# CHAPTER ONE

# Introduction

Health Information Technology[1] (HIT) is receiving attention from the U.S. President on down, and many would like to see it play an expanded role in providing care. The result of our effort to gain a better understanding of the potential of HIT to transform the provision of healthcare is documented in Hillestad et al. (2005), and the policy implications of that work are reported in Taylor et al. (2005). In this monograph, we expand on some of the quantitative aspects of the Hillestad et al. and Taylor et al. research, providing detailed supporting material on the following four related aspects of that research:

- **Extrapolation of savings to the national level and projection of savings into the future (Chapter Two):** The research in Hillestad et al. (2005) focuses on the benefits and costs that would accrue to and be sustained by the nation as a whole as a result of widespread adoption of HIT. Our first step is to provide a methodological framework to scale empirical evidence on the effect of HIT at the national level and to project it into the future. A key element of this framework is a projection for the rates of adoption of HIT in the inpatient setting and in the ambulatory/outpatient setting. This component is developed using models of HIT adoption and analysis of historical data found in Bower (2005) and Fonkych and Taylor (2005) and in work developed by Hillestad, Taylor, and others as part of the same project. Projections of HIT adoption can then be combined with data on specific effects of HIT at the provider level and on national expenditures to provide projections of future national savings in certain health sectors.

---

[1] We use Health Information Technology (HIT) and Electronic Medical Record System (EMR-S) interchangeably in this report. An EMR-S, as we use it here, includes the Electronic Medical Record (EMR), which contains current and historical patient information; Clinical Decision Support (CDS), which provides reminders and best-practice guidance for treatment; and a Central Data Repository, which stores the EMR information. It also includes information technology–enabled functions, such as Computerized Physician Order Entry (CPOE), which facilitates orders tied to patient-information and -treatment pathways.

Clearly the methodology developed in this chapter is useless without a set of empirical findings. Therefore, we also document in this chapter the extensive literature search we performed, seeking evidence on the effects of HIT at the provider level. Unfortunately, much of the available evidence is incomplete and cannot be scaled to the national level because key measures are lacking—only 42 findings being extracted from the more than 1,400 articles we screened.

- **Benefits of HIT (Chapter Three):** The benefits we focus on in this document are the efficiency savings that are enabled by HIT, whereas the HIT-related benefits discussed in Bigelow et al. (2005b) are in health improvement. In this context, *efficiency savings* are what results from the ability to perform the same task with fewer resources (money, time, personnel, etc.). From the evidence found by the literature search, we consider savings from 10 different sources: five for the inpatient sector (such as savings coming from reduction in length of stay or increases in nurses' productivity) and five for the outpatient/ambulatory sector (such as reduction in transcription costs or drug expenditures). For each of these sources, we detail the nature of the data and the extrapolation procedure and report the *potential savings*—that is, the savings that would accrue if the HIT adoption rate were to jump to 100 percent overnight—as well as the mean yearly savings over the next 15 years.

- **Costs of HIT (Chapter Four):** The efficiency savings documented in Chapter Three need to be compared with the costs the nation has to incur in order to be able to realize those savings. We estimated these costs using a modeling framework analogous to the one developed for the extrapolation of savings. Our cost data were gathered through the literature or given to us by providers during site visits.

The RAND Corporation team made about 15 site visits to a variety of healthcare institutions—large healthcare systems, teaching hospitals, regional health networks, and research organizations associated with medical centers. Most of the sites already had some form of EMR-S or were in the process of acquiring an EMR-S. Within each site, the RAND team interviewed physicians, nurses, hospital managers, administrators, and researchers, enabling us to look at EMR-S from the viewpoint of different occupations. The multiplicity of sites allowed us to observe EMR-S at different stages of development and/or built for different purposes.

Site visits were also used to gather relevant data, which were provided either informally, as expert opinion, or as a set of actual observations (EMR-S cost data, for example). The information gained from the site visits was supplemented with literally hundreds of conference calls and phone conversations with a disparate set of individuals—leaders of physician and hospital associations, EMR-S vendors, EMR-S users, researchers in the field of healthcare organization and healthcare information technology, academics, and government officials. The results of these site visits and conference calls form a body of knowledge from which we extracted both a vision of the current status of EMR-S and some of the data we have used in this monograph.

- **Incentives for Adoption of HIT (Chapter Five):** Even a cursory look at benefits and costs shows that the savings enabled by widespread HIT adoption are significantly larger than the expenditures on EMR-S that would have to be incurred in order for those savings to materialize. If we aggregate over all healthcare sectors, we project mean annual savings of almost $42 billion, while mean annual costs are about $7.6 billion. Obviously, these numbers would be larger if the adoption of HIT happened at a faster rate than is projected. Therefore, we studied what might be the effect of those financial incentives presented to providers that lower the cost of EMR-S and quicken the pace of HIT adoption. In particular, we considered per-encounter payments to physicians who adopt an EMR-S and percentage subsidies to hospitals. The estimation of costs and benefits of such incentives is especially difficult, because it requires us to know how sensitive providers are to the price of EMR-S, something that has never been measured. Despite this uncertainty, we relied on sensitivity analysis to conclude that, even under pessimistic assumptions, programs aimed at incentivizing HIT adoption can deliver benefits that outweigh costs.

The chapters outlined above are followed by a summary chapter. Readers interested in the policy issues related to HIT adoption and/or desiring to put this document in a more general perspective are encouraged to read Hillestad et al. (2005) and Taylor et al. (2005).

Throughout this document, we refer to a number of Excel spreadsheets that contain additional information and allow the user to interact with some of our models. The spreadsheets are part of the online monograph at http://www.rand.org/publications/MG/MG410 and are cited by their file names.

# CHAPTER TWO

# Scaling Up and Projecting Savings into the Future

## Typical Scenario for National-Level Savings

Our typical scenario for how we use evidence from the literature on HIT-related savings to extrapolate the savings figures to the national level involves a provider (a physician or a hospital) that incurs a yearly expenditure of a certain type and uses HIT to reduce it. We refer to the yearly expenditure per provider as the *base cost B,* and we denote the percentage reduction (savings) in base cost obtained by using HIT as *s*. For example, a physician might buy an EMR-S and be able to save 50 percent (*s*=0.5) of his or her yearly expenditure of $7,000 (*B*=7,000) on transcription services. The parameter *s* is usually derived by averaging several findings from the literature; *B* is usually obtained from a variety of sources on health care expenditure, such as the National Health Expenditures (NHE) (Centers for Medicare & Medicaid Services, 2005a), or physician and hospital associations.

If *N* is the national number of providers, then in year *t* the savings at the national level is

$$S_t = sBNp_t, \qquad (2.1)$$

where $p_t$ is the adoption rate in year *t*—that is, the proportion of people who have adopted an EMR-S by year *t*. Note that $p_t$ is a cumulative measure; it should not be confused with the proportion of providers who adopt *in* year *t*, which is equal to $p_t - p_{t-1}$. *For the purpose of this section, we assume that there is no significant delay between adoption of HIT and the realization of savings; we consider the case with a delay in the following subsection, "Duration of Implementation and Delayed Savings."* The product *sBN* is a recurring quantity in this document, and we refer to it as the "base savings."

The quantity $S_t$ above, however, is not useful for policy purposes, since it includes "sunk" savings, savings that have accrued to providers who have adopted already. More specifically, since we performed this study during the year 2004, we do not want to include in our calculations the savings to providers who adopted before or during the year 2004. Therefore, we define the savings at the national level as

$$S_t \equiv sBN(p_t - p_{2004}), \qquad (2.2)$$

where $S_t$=0 for $t$<2004. Definition (2.2) is what we will use for $S_t$ in the rest of this section. According to this definition, if the adoption rate $p_t$ flattened out in year 2004, the projected savings would always be zero. This is a reasonable assumption, because we wish to quantify the savings due to the *increased* level of HIT with respect to the status quo. The value of $p_{2004}$ varies with the setting (inpatient or outpatient), and it is discussed in Chapter Three.

The savings projections above depend on the projections for the adoption rate $p_t$ (the adoption curve). In this monograph, we use the adoption curve derived by Bower (2005), which is governed by the following difference equation:

$$p_{t+1} = p_t + bp_t(m - p_t). \qquad (2.3)$$

The parameter $b$ is often referred as the *adoption speed,* and it is related to the *adoption time* $T_{10 \to 90}$, which we define as the time it takes for the adoption rate to go from 10 percent to 90 percent, by the formula:

$$b = \frac{2\log(9)}{T_{10 \to 90}}. \qquad (2.4)$$

To set the value of $b$, we use Bower's analysis (2005), in which he concludes that IT in healthcare is expected to diffuse at a pace similar to that of a large-scale relational database or mainframe computer (the so-called Cluster 2 technologies in the terminology of Tang, Grover, and Guttler [2002]). For such technologies, the adoption speed $b$ has been, on average, 0.3, corresponding to an adoption time of about 15 years. A more direct way to estimate $b$ is from empirical adoption curves, which can be computed, for example, from the Dorenfest database (Health Information Management System Society [HIMSS], second release, 2004) (formerly the Dorenfest IHDS+TM Database), which contains longitudinal information on all integrated healthcare delivery systems[1] in the United States. Using the empirical adoption curves computed in Fonkych and Taylor (2005), we also find that the

---

[1] An *integrated healthcare delivery system* is a network of healthcare providers and organizations that provides or arranges to provide a continuum of services to a defined population and is clinically and fiscally accountable for the clinical outcomes and health status of the population served.

parameter $b$ is about 0.3; therefore, we set $b=0.3$ in our computations. In our sensitivity analysis, we use values of $b$ that correspond to adoption times of 10 and 20 years.

The parameter $m$ is the asymptotic value of the adoption rate, which we take to be 1, assuming that, in the long term, eventually everybody will adopt some sort of EMR-S. There is clearly no evidence to support this statement, which we take mostly as a simplifying assumption.

Since savings are characterized as a function of time, it is convenient to introduce a few summary measures of savings:

- **Potential savings:** The potential savings PS are the yearly savings that will be realized once adoption reaches 100 percent. Formally, they are

$$PS \equiv sBN(1 - p_{2004}). \tag{2.5}$$

  Equivalently, these are the yearly savings that would be realized if all the providers who have not adopted an EMR-S adopted one instantly in year 2005.
- **Cumulative savings:** Let $T$ be a fixed time horizon. The cumulative savings $CS(T)$ defined below are useful to quantify how much better the country is after $T$ years of increased adoption rates:

$$CS(T) \equiv \sum_{t=2004}^{2004+T-1} S_t. \tag{2.6}$$

Note that the sum has $T$ terms and that the first term is always 0 because there are no savings in the year 2004.[2] A discounting rate $r$ can be introduced, leading to a modification of Equation (2.6) as follows:

$$CS(T) \equiv \sum_{t=2004}^{2004+T-1} w_t S_t, \tag{2.7}$$

where $w_t=(1+r)^{-(t-2004)}$. Note that here $r$ is the interest rate minus the growth rate of healthcare expenditures. We have chosen to use the value of $r=0$ in our calculations, assuming that the interest rate and the growth rate of healthcare expenditures cancel each other. This is a conservative assumption, which may understate the cumulative savings. In fact, for the past two decades, healthcare expenditures have been increasing at rates that are, on average, higher than in-

---

[2] A different, more transparent notation would have been preferable. We maintain this notation here for consistency with other parts of this project, which started in 2003.

terest rates. This disparity can be seen in Figure 2.1, where we plot on the same graph the annual percentage increase in national health expenditures and the nominal interest rate, measured by the 10-year Treasury constant-maturity yield. We can see that, on average, healthcare expenditures increase at a rate that is 1 percentage point higher than the nominal interest rate.

• **Mean yearly savings**: These are simple averages obtained by dividing the cumulative savings by the time horizon $T$:

$$\text{MYS}(T) \equiv \frac{1}{T} \sum_{t=2004}^{2004+T-1} S_t. \tag{2.8}$$

Note that there is no discounting in this formula. If we assume a discount rate $r$, then the formula would be modified as follows:

$$\text{MYS}(T) \equiv \frac{\displaystyle\sum_{t=2004}^{2004+T-1} w_t S_t}{\displaystyle\sum_{t=2004}^{2004+T-1} w_t}, \tag{2.9}$$

where $w_t = (1+r)^{-(t-2004)}$. According to this formula, the mean yearly savings is the constant yearly figure whose discounted sum over $T$ periods is equal to the discounted cumulative savings.

It is very important to notice that *mean yearly savings are usually about half the potential savings*. This is an empirical finding that does not depend on the size of the savings and will become clear once we start looking at specific results. The reason for this independence is related to the current (low) rate of adoption and the fact that the time horizon $T$ is 15 years, the same as the adoption time $T_{10\rightarrow90}$ (clearly if $T \gg T_{10\rightarrow90}$, potential savings and mean yearly savings would be very similar). The difference between mean yearly savings and potential savings is a useful reminder that savings occur over time and that the potential savings will be realized only when, and if, adoption reaches 100 percent.

• **Savings in/by year $t$**: In some of our tables, we also report the yearly savings in or by year $t$ after the baseline year (where "by" means that cumulative savings are computed). The baseline year is 2004 unless otherwise specified. Typical choices for $t$ are 5, 10, and 15. Another option is to report savings in/by the year in which adoption reaches a certain level (for example, savings by adoption at 90 percent means the cumulative savings from 2004 to year 2018, the year in which adoption is expected to reach 90 percent). This last definition should be used with care, because it computes savings over a time interval whose size changes with the parameters of the adoption curve.

**Figure 2.1**
**Nominal Interest Rate, Measured by the 10-Year Treasury Constant-Maturity Yield\*, and Medical Care Inflation, Measured by the Annual Percentage Increase in National Health Expenditures\*\***

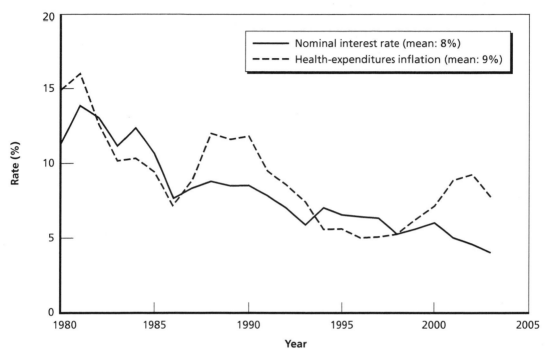

SOURCES: Authors' calculations
\*Obtained from http://www.federalreserve.gov/Releases/H15/data.htm
\*\*Obtained from Centers for Medicare & Medicaid Services, 2005a
**RAND** *MG410-2.1*

Note that estimating the national savings requires the *product* of the three quantities, *s, B,* and *N.* We see in the rest of the monograph that, although the individual terms of the product are sometimes not known, potential savings can still be computed. For example, we may know that a certain intervention saves *s* percent of a hospital's operating expenses. Then, all we need to know is the national level of hospital operating expenses—the product *BN*—which is easier to find than the total number of hospitals *N* and the average hospital operating expense *B*. We refer to the quantity *BN* as the *national-level base cost.* Similarly, findings in the literature may tell us that a certain intervention leads to a certain amount of dollars saved per physician, which can be seen as the product *sB;* then, all we need to know is the total number of physicians in the United States.

### Duration of Implementation and Delayed Savings
The pattern of savings over time described in the preceding section assumes that savings accrue to the adopter in the same year as the adoption. In practice, it may

take a few years to implement an EMR-S (especially in the inpatient setting), and, therefore, there might be a delay between the beginning of the implementation and the time the full savings are realized, with only partial savings realized during the implementation phase. If we want to take this delay into account, we have to be precise in our definition of adoption rate $p_t$. In the following discussion, we define $p_t$ as the percentage of providers who, by year $t$, have *completed* the implementation phase, of duration $\tau$.[3] When $\tau = 1$, the EMR-S is implemented within a year from the beginning of the implementation phase: There is no delay between adoption and savings and the adoption rate $p_t$ coincides with the adoption rate defined in the preceding section. When $\tau = 2$, it takes two years to implement the EMR-S, and therefore in this case $p_t$ is the percentage of providers who have started to implement the EMR-S in year $t-1$ or earlier. In general, $p_t$ is equal to the percentage of providers who have started to implement their EMR-S in year $t-\tau+1$ or earlier. Note that $\tau = 1$ corresponds to the case of no delay.

To model this pattern of savings, we make the assumption that savings increase linearly during the implementation phase. Therefore, if the implementation time is $\tau$ years, and if the savings at the end of the implementation will be $S$, then $S/\tau$ is saved in the first year, $2S/\tau$ is saved in the second year, and $S$ is saved from the $\tau$-th year on. Under this assumption, Equation (2.1) must be replaced by the following:

$$S_t(\tau) = \frac{sBN}{\tau} \sum_{k=1}^{\tau} p_{t+k-1}. \tag{2.10}$$

Note that the savings in year $t$ depend on future values of the adoption rate, because there are fractions of savings accruing to providers who start to implement in year $t$, but those providers are not counted as adopters until $\tau$ years later. This fact depends only on our definition of $p_t$, which does not include providers who are just starting to adopt. Equation (2.10) does not take in account the fact that we want to subtract the savings of those who decided to adopt in or by 2004. An easy way to account for this subtraction is to define a "counterfactual" profile of adoption $\hat{p}_t$, obtained by assuming that no new providers decide to adopt after the year 2004 (although those who started during, or before, will complete their implementation). Then, the definition of savings is modified by subtracting from Equation (2.10) the pattern of savings that would be obtained if the profile $\hat{p}_t$ occurred, instead of $p_t$:

---

[3] We make the assumption that providers always complete the implementation once they start.

$$S_t(\tau) = \frac{sBN}{\tau} \sum_{k=1}^{\tau} (p_{t+k-1} - \hat{p}_{t+k-1}). \qquad (2.11)$$

It is easy to verify that if $\tau=1$, this definition coincides with the one in Equation (2.2), since in this case $\hat{p}_t = p_{2004}$ for $t>2004$. All the definitions given in the preceding section still apply, although the final expressions as a function of $p_t$ obviously differ. The formula for the potential savings given in Equation (2.5) now takes a particularly simple form, as shown in Equation (2.12):

$$PS(\tau) \equiv sBN(1 - p_{2004+\tau-1}). \qquad (2.12)$$

In this formula, the term $p_{2004+\tau-1}$ represents the savings of those who *decided* to adopt prior to the year 2004 (included). It is useful to note that the yearly savings can be expressed as a function of the potential savings. In fact, we can use Equation (2.12) to rewrite Equation (2.11), as follows:

$$S_t(\tau) = \frac{PS(\tau)}{\tau(1 - p_{2004+\tau-1})} \sum_{k=1}^{\tau} (p_{t+k-1} - \hat{p}_{t+k-1}). \qquad (2.13)$$

Therefore the time evolution of the savings is uniquely determined by the potential savings, the delay $\tau$, and the adoption curve, a fact that will be used in the "Summary of Savings at the National Level" section of Chapter Three.

The potential savings are clearly a decreasing function of $\tau$; therefore, longer delays will lead to smaller values of the potential savings. However, since the current adoption rate is fairly low (15–20 percent) and the adoption time is fairly long (15 years), the potential savings vary very little with $\tau$. Using the adoption curve of Equation (2.3), it is easy to show that the percentage difference between the potential savings corresponding to adjacent values of $\tau$ is as follows:

$$\frac{PS(\tau) - PS(\tau+1)}{PS(\tau)} = bp_{2004+\tau-1}. \qquad (2.14)$$

For $\tau=1$, with the standard values of $b=0.3$ and $p_{2004}=0.15$, the product above is 0.045.

Similarly to the potential savings, cumulative and mean yearly savings are also a decreasing function of $\tau$, since they sum over a time period during which savings are 0, because they still accrue to "old adopters."

To give the reader an idea of how much the cumulative and yearly savings change with the parameter $\tau$, we report in Figure 2.2 the cumulative savings for increasing values of $\tau$ for the case in which the product $sBN$ is such that the cumulative savings over 15 years with no delay is $1 billion. With an implementation time of $\tau=4$, the cumulative savings are at $0.88 billion—that is, 12 percent less than those with $\tau=1$.

We are then left with the choice of $\tau$ for the inpatient setting and the outpatient setting. For the outpatient setting, we chose $\tau=2$, based on limited evidence and our interviews with experts in this area. The best-documented evidence comes from a practice with nine full-time equivalent employees (FTEs) (Roswell Pediatric Center, 2003), which represents a best-case scenario, because it received the Davies Award for Primary Care, a yearly award given to organizations that excel in health information management. This practice purchased the system in August 2001 and started using it in November 2001, reaping its benefits gradually over six months from the moment it went live. Although we do not have such detailed data for all the recipients of the Davies Award, many of them suggest an implementation phase of one year, with a

**Figure 2.2**
**Cumulative Savings as a Function of the Parameter $\tau$.**

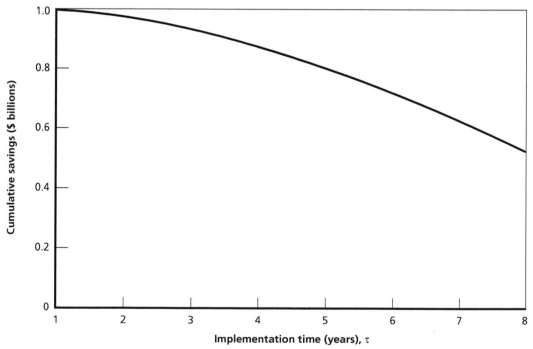

NOTE: $\tau=1$ means implementation takes 1 year, and therefore savings are realized at the end of that year, so it corresponds to 0 year of delay.
RAND *MG410-2.2*

very rapid learning curve (Pediatrics @ the Basin, 2004; Riverpoint Pediatrics, 2004; North Fulton Family Medicine, 2004; Old Harding Pediatrics Associates, 2004; Cooper Pediatrics, 2003). This evidence points to a value of $\tau$ equal to 1.

While not all the practices that adopt an EMR-S are award winners and might not have the same success, other sources of evidence point at an implementation phase of about one year. For example, many of the savings figures that we use were obtained by comparing costs at two points in time, separated by a year (sometimes less), and we did find several references explicitly quoting a year as the time it takes to see some results (CCA Medical, 2005; Sandrick, 1998; MedicaLogic, 2004; Pifer et al., 2001; Cap Gemini Ernst & Young, 2004). Consistent with our general strategy of being conservative and representing neither a best-case scenario nor a worst-case scenario, we decided to use a value of $\tau=2$.

For hospitals, we chose a value of $\tau$ equal to 4. This figure is mostly based on the detailed project time line provided to us by a large hospital system that implemented a fairly sophisticated EMR-S, and on conversations with hospital executives who have detailed knowledge of the implementation process. There are several reasons we expect this figure to decrease with time, although we do not take this possibility into account in our model, in order to remain conservative. One is that the hospital market in the United States is dominated by small hospitals (around 100 beds), and smaller hospitals are more likely to adopt application service providers (ASP) delivery models, which do not require installation of much infrastructure and tend to lead to lower implementation time. Another reason is that we expect vendors to learn over time and become quicker in their implementation. An example of such learning is GE Healthcare, which took 18 months for the installation and implementation of an EMR-S (with such features as CPOE, Picture Archiving Communications Systems (PACS), Clinical Decision Support, and electronic patient records) at the 50-bed Indiana Heart Hospital in Indianapolis, and only 9 months for its subsequent installation at the similarly sized Saint Francis Heart Hospital in Tulsa, Oklahoma (Versel, 2004). We also expect to see a quickening of the pace at which physicians are trained in the hospital. One hospital executive we interviewed noted that younger cohorts of physicians are becoming increasingly comfortable with computer technology and, therefore, do not require as much training as older cohorts.

For the above reasons, we assign $\tau=2$ for the outpatient setting and $\tau=4$ for the inpatient setting. Using Figure 2.2, readers can quickly compute what the effect on cumulative savings of changing the value $\tau$ would be. To allow readers to get a feel for how the other parameters of our model affect the computations of the savings, we have provided the interactive Excel spreadsheet ambulatory_savings_simulator.xls, which simulates the scenario in which a physician can save $s$ percent of his or her base cost $B$ and allows the user to choose interactively the parameters of the adoption curve, the percentage saved $s$, the base cost $B$, the number of physicians $N$, and the time horizon $T$. As these parameters vary, the users can observe changes in the adoption curve and the yearly savings curve given by Equation (2.11), as well as in the mean yearly savings and the potential savings.

## Literature Search and Empirical Findings on Savings

The modeling framework described in the preceding section relies on the availability of a key parameter, the percentage savings $s$. Therefore, we performed an extensive literature search for studies that quantified the value of specific interventions supported by HIT. Here, we report key features and findings of this search.

We assumed that the available literature would be abundant and that findings would be easily identified at the level we needed to support the development of our models. Because of the anticipated volume of articles and the rapidly changing health technology market, we limited the primary search to systematic reviews and meta-analyses from the years 1995 through 2004. After screening these articles for relevance, we scanned their reference lists to identify prior articles that would be informative, salient, and contain scalable data. However, we recognized that the gray literature (the body of reports and studies produced by local government agencies, private organizations, and educational facilities, which have not been reviewed and published in journals or other standard research publications) also contained a plethora of information that was being published continuously due to the ever-increasing use of HIT. As a result, we included five components in the search (Table 2.1). Some interesting and differentiating characteristics appeared between the two primary types of literature, as defined in Table 2.2.

The modeling effort required identifying specific empirical evidence of the quantitative effect of HIT on a process or outcome measure (a "finding"). The evidence also had to be attached to a specific segment of the healthcare system and a particular technologic intervention so that it could be appropriately scaled for other segments (e.g., academic medical centers, general acute care hospitals, physician offices). To accomplish this categorization, we developed three taxonomies that permitted us to classify the effects the technology had on one or more of the Institute of Medicine's (IOM, 2001) six aims for quality, what type of interventions were used, and what features or functions of HIT were employed. The taxonomies are described in Appendix A. The majority of evidence was collected from the peer-reviewed literature.

All relevant articles were screened by one of the analysts or research assistants on the research team, using a one-page form (short form) providing information on the research topic, general type of intervention employed, type of information technol-

**Table 2.1**
**Components of the Literature Search**

| | Type of Literature | Years | Search Strategy | Number of Articles |
|---|---|---|---|---|
| 1) | Peer-reviewed literature—systematic reviews and meta-analyses | 1995–2004 | Peer-reviewed publications identified through PubMed, CINAHL | 1,107 retrieved from database scans |
| | | | Major Headings—medical, health, informatics, electronic (and related combinations), AND Systematic AND Cost, outcome | 347 relevant articles |
| | | | | 63 systematic reviews |
| | | | | 36 reviews snowballed for articles |
| | | | | 19 additional articles searched for findings |
| 2) | Literature snowballed from systematic reviews and meta-analyses | >1980 | | 285 articles snowballed |
| | | | | 90 articles searched for findings |
| 3) | Gray literature—HIT journals, conference proceedings, government reports, healthcare trade journals | 2000–2004 | Scanned tables of contents and websites for relevant items | More than 2,000 items scanned |
| | | | | 222 articles screened |
| | | | | 64 articles searched for findings |
| 4) | Topic-specific searches | 2002–2004 | MEDLINE searches focused on specific HIT topics of interest to the project: e.g., quality improvement, disease management | 355 articles retrieved from database scans |
| | | | | 153 relevant articles |
| | | | | 17 searched for findings |
| 5) | Additional snowballs, recommended articles | | | 32 articles searched for findings |
| | Articles searched for findings | | | 222 |
| | Articles that yielded findings | | | 202 |

NOTE: The primary search of the peer-reviewed literature was limited to articles published in the years 1995 through 2004 (row 1). Articles snowballed from that search (row 2) may date from before the year 1995.

**Table 2.2**
**Differentiating Characteristics of Peer-Reviewed and Gray Literature**

| Characteristic | Peer-Reviewed | Gray |
| --- | --- | --- |
| Audience | Providers, academics, informaticists | Corporate information officers (CIOs), technical staff, implementers |
| Focus | Clinical processes and outcomes | Economic return |
| Content | Is based on experimental design; has good description of measures | Project descriptions and case studies; often poor description of measures and returns |
| Type of findings | Improved appropriate care for patients; reduced errors and costs | Reduced costs, increased revenues |

ogy utilized, design of the study, care setting, patient population, article origin, and, if the article was rejected, the reason for the rejection. Articles with empirical evidence were then screened by two analysts, using an extensive form (long form) that required a detailed description of the care setting, each of the taxonomies, and a quantitative description of the findings at a level that could be applied to a model of the healthcare system. All short-form and long-form information was recorded in an Access database. The database permitted the team to identify interventions for which no findings had been identified through the formal search and gray literature. Among other things, this step informed the fourth level of the literature review: topic-specific searches that were not always HIT-specific—e.g., disease management and quality improvement.

The database was then used to identify relevant and scalable[4] preliminary findings to be included in the models. We found that much of the available evidence for the impact of HIT is limited, ambiguous, incomplete, and inconclusive. For example, in many publications a savings figure was provided in absolute terms, but no information was available to convert it to a percentage savings. Consequently, some peer-reviewed literature passed the initial short-form screen but was of marginal value to the project goals; therefore, it was not evaluated.

In total, 1,418 articles were screened using the short form, and 202 articles were coded according to taxonomies, yielding 581 preliminary findings, of which 42 were ultimately included in the models as defined below in Table 2.3. The reason that many findings were not used in our models is that they were not scalable: The key quantities necessary to scale the finding to the national level were missing. For

---

[4] A finding is *scalable* if it can be used to extrapolate savings to the national level.

**Table 2.3**
**Findings by Topic**

| Total Preliminary Findings | 581 | |
|---|---|---|
| Findings Within Topic Areas | Preliminary | Scalable |
| Transcriptions | 14 | 11 |
| Paper-record savings | 17 | 12 |
| Reduced nursing time | 27 | 3 |
| Reduced lab tests (inpatient) | 7 | 2 |
| Reduced lab tests (outpatient) | 5 | 3 |
| Reduced drug costs (inpatient) | 10 | 1 |
| Reduced drug costs (outpatient) | 13 | 6 |
| Radiology | 8 | 1 |
| Reduction in length of stay | 8 | 3 |

example, we may find in the literature that introduction of EMR-S may lead to reductions in a particular type of laboratory test, providing us a figure for the percentage savings $s$. However, if we do not know how many of these tests are performed nationally and how much they cost, this finding is useless ("not scalable"). Similarly, we may find that a HIT intervention leads to a reduced turnaround time for radiology tests, but it may be impossible to translate such a finding into a dollar amount.

# CHAPTER THREE

# Estimating the Benefits of HIT

In this chapter, we set out to quantify the benefits of HIT by extrapolating findings from the literature to the national level. We document savings separately for the inpatient sector and the outpatient sector, where by *outpatient* we mean all the ambulatory practices, and not necessarily only those associated with hospitals. (Other transaction and administrative costs relating to claims processing and insurance-program enrollment are discussed in Appendix B.) Within each sector, we consider several categories of savings, such as the savings related to reductions in duplicate laboratory tests or to reductions in length of stay. For each category of savings, we report the details of the extrapolation procedure, together with the potential and mean savings. To keep the document readable, the individual findings on the effect of HIT, the sources of those findings, and sources for additional data used to compute the base cost are reported in the Excel spreadsheets savings_inpatient.xls and savings_outpaticnt.xls available onlinc at the same website of this document. For each finding we also report the type of study (randomized control trial, or pre/post, for example), the setting (family practice, large urban hospital, . . . ) and the type of publication (peer-reviewed, conference proceedings, . . . ). This additional information is meant to allow readers to judge for themselves the validity and reliability of the evidence used in this document. These spreadsheets contain one worksheet for each savings category, as well as a worksheet named "Source list" with the entire list of sources analyzed in the literature search (more than 1,400 entries). A summary of the evidence used for the extrapolation, with all the findings on percentage savings in one single worksheet, is in the spreadsheet summary_of_evidence.xls.

Readers not interested in the details of the calculations can go directly to Table 3.2 at the end of this chapter, in which we summarize our findings. In that table, we report, for each savings category, the potential savings, the mean yearly savings, the cumulative savings, and the savings at years 5, 10, and 15 from the base year, 2004. Unless otherwise specified, all the dollar amounts appearing in this document are in 2004 dollars.

Some important parameters are necessary to extrapolate the findings:

- **The number of physicians:** For our purposes, we need the number of non-institutional, non-federal, post-GME (Graduate Medical Education) practicing physicians. We chose the non-institutional physicians because we do not wish to include providers working in hospitals (to avoid double-counting with the inpatient setting) and universities or local government offices (since these settings are not in our universe of findings). The number of non-institutional physicians is not reported in the most recent publication on physician statistics (American Medical Association, 2005, for the year 2003), but is given as 413,280 in Kane (2004) for the year 2001. For our extrapolation, we wished to use the corresponding number for 2005, which is not available. Therefore, we used the rate of growth in the total number of physicians in patient care to estimate its value, which turns out to be 442,104. Note that the number for 2001 will be used in some additional computations in the following section; because it will appear in the context of data referring to the past few years, it is more appropriate.

- **Initial adoption rate $p_{2001}$:** A number of surveys and studies report adoption rates for HIT; a review of such literature can be found in Fonkych and Taylor (2005). However, survey results are often difficult to interpret, for several reasons. One is that there is no consistent definition of EMR-S in the literature. For the purpose of our exercise, we need the percentage of providers who, in the year 2004, have an EMR-S in place with all the capabilities required to achieve the type of efficiency savings we address; therefore, our definition of EMR-S is fairly restrictive. For example, in the 2003 Commonwealth Fund National Survey of Physicians and Quality of Care, which randomly samples U.S. physicians, 21 percent of physicians reported using a computerized system for patient reminders, but only 6 percent routinely used electronic Clinical Decision Support, and only 10 percent routinely used computerized systems for follow-up alert (Audet et al., 2004). In addition, many surveys reported in the literature are likely to overestimate the adoption of HIT, either because physicians in their sample are more likely to have an EMR-S or because physicians who have an EMR-S have more incentives to respond to such surveys. The most complete survey on the state of HIT adoption is the Dorenfest database (HIMSS, 2004), which contains information on all integrated healthcare delivery systems in the nation.

  For ambulatory practices, the analysis of the Dorenfest database described in Fonkych and Taylor (2005) and Bower (2005) suggests an initial adoption rate in 2004 of around 15 percent. This percentage is consistent with the physicians' data from the Commonwealth Fund described in Audet et al. (2004), if we take figures referring to routine use of IT (excluding occasional use, which does not fit our purposes). An extensive analysis of adoption patterns of HIT among hospitals, mostly based on the Dorenfest database, is presented in Fonkych and

Taylor (2005), where estimates of current adoption rates are provided for several definitions of EMR-S. Using their most conservative definitions of EMR-S, we conclude from that analysis that a reasonable estimate for the current adoption rate is 20 percent. We use these values throughout this document, with excursions of ±5 percentage points in our sensitivity analysis.

- **Adoption curve parameters:** For the adoption curve, we use an adoption time of 15 years and an asymptotic value of adoption $m=1$, as discussed in Chapter Two.
- **Implementation time:** The delay parameter $\tau$ is 2 years and 4 years for the outpatient and inpatient settings, respectively, as discussed in Chapter Two.

## Outpatient

Many findings in the literature document HIT-related savings in many areas of the ambulatory setting; however, not all of them can be extrapolated to the national level, usually because they are too specific or because crucial data needed for the extrapolation are missing. In five areas of intervention, data are sufficient for the extrapolation, providing a lower bound for the size of the savings that could be realized by the widespread adoption of ambulatory EMR-S: transcription, chart pulls, laboratory tests, drug utilization, and radiology/imaging.

### Transcription

Physicians frequently rely on dictation as a fast way to record notes of both inpatient and outpatient encounters. Audio tapes or digital audio files are typically transcribed by a service outside the physician's office. The record is then approved and signed by the physician before it is inserted into the chart. The process is widely acknowledged to be expensive, slow, inefficient, and prone to error. Transcription, in principle, can be eliminated when clinicians enter notes directly into an EMR-S. Variations include entering notes in the exam room with the patient present or using a system-generated summary sheet during the visit, then entering data after the patient has departed. Encounter templates—in some cases, touchscreens—or summary sheets can be structured according to the patient's condition or the nature of the visit (for example, annual exam versus trauma, male versus female, and so on). It is not uncommon during the transition to an EMR-S for clinicians to use dictation for some types of encounters and direct entry of notes for others, or, in a group practice or hospital, for some providers to switch to direct notes entry while others continue with dictation.

**Percentage Savings.** Most of the 11 literature findings about savings in transcription costs report the percentage savings. Only one finding gave an absolute number for the savings: a urologist/pediatrician who saved $600 per month in transcription costs (MacDonald and Metzger, 2002). From the *2003 Cost Survey* performed by the Medical Group Management Association (MGMA, http://www .mgma.com/surveys/index.cfm), we found that urologists, after taking into account employee benefits, spend an average of $13,900 per year on transcription, which equals $1,158 per month. Savings of $600 are then equivalent to a reduction in transcription cost of 48 percent. We added this figure to the other 10 found in the literature and obtained an average savings of 73.5 percent.

**Extrapolation of Savings.** From our calculations based on the MGMA *2003 Physicians Cost Survey,* the average practice spends $7,094 per year per FTE on transcription costs. This value includes allocated employee benefits, and it should be compared with the $5,891 per year in 2001 published by MGMA (Moore, 2002), which, once adjusted for inflation to 2004 dollars, becomes $6,240. It is our understanding that the MGMA figure does not include employee benefits, whereas our figure does. Since employee benefits should be included, we prefer to use the figure from our calculations.

**National Savings.** Based on the figures reported above, we estimated that the potential savings from reductions in transcription cost are $1.9 billion, corresponding to mean yearly savings of $0.9 billion and cumulative savings over 15 years of $13.4 billion.

## Chart Pulls

EMR-S reduce or eliminate the need to maintain paper patient files. A number of savings accrue: There will be no need to fetch or refile a paper chart for office visits or other transactions, and no time will be wasted looking for misplaced charts. Once its patient data are in electronic form, a practice can recoup resources related to chart handling and maintenance: personnel costs, supplies, and the opportunity cost represented by the physical space devoted to chart storage, which can be eliminated or turned to revenue-producing activities. In addition, there is a reduction or elimination in supplies, copying fees, and, for some sites, off-site storage costs. However, these gains are not automatic: An EMR-S–equipped practice will still receive paper documents in the form of lab reports, referral letters, and so on. Some practices scan these into the patient's EMR and shred the originals. Because the document need only be handled once, and because the scanning process itself is relatively fast, overall personnel costs for handling a document can be reduced. EMR-S–equipped practices that do not scan must maintain their patient files to store paper documents.

**Percentage Savings.** Many results from the literature are given in terms of the percentage reduction in the number of charts pulled by each practice. We make the assumption that the percentage reduction in chart pulls is matched by an equal percentage reduction in the number of medical records clerks. Other data are given directly in terms of percentage reduction in medical records clerks. Combining all these findings, we obtained an estimated savings of 63.4 percent in expenditures on medical records personnel.

**Extrapolation of Savings.** Using the MGMA *2003 Cost Survey* data, we estimated that the average practice spends $7,345 per FTE on medical records. This number, which includes employee benefits, is in very good agreement with the $6,783 figure given by MGMA in 2001 (Moore, 2002), which, adjusted for inflation to 2004 dollars, becomes $7,185.

**Validation.** Here, we validate the figure of $7,345 in yearly expenditures per FTE on medical records with an alternative calculation. A reasonable estimate of the time involved in each chart pull is about 4 minutes. The number of chart pulls per physician per day is larger than the number of visits by a factor 1.6 (for example, because of telephone contacts between physician and patients) (Bingham, 1997). With an average of 15 patients per day per physician, 5 days a week for 48 weeks, we estimate 5,760 chart pulls per year per physician, which amounts to 384 hours of staff time. According to the National Compensation Survey of the Bureau of Labor Statistics (http://www.bls.gov/ncs/home.htm), the average hourly cost to the employer of service personnel in healthcare and social assistance jobs is $14.4, which leads to an estimated expenditure on medical records personnel of $5,530 per year.

**National Savings.** From the figures reported above, we estimated that the potential savings from reduction in chart pulls are $1.7 billion, corresponding to mean yearly savings of $0.8 billion and cumulative savings over 15 years of $11.9 billion.

## Laboratory Tests

When patients are seen by multiple providers, either in an inpatient setting or across multiple care settings, orders for redundant diagnostic tests may occur simply because providers are unaware of the results of tests ordered by others. In other cases, tests may be ordered that are not germane to a patient's principal complaint, but because of habit, personal preference, etc. In an evaluation of 10 common inpatient diagnostic tests, Bates and Boyle (1998) estimated that 8.6 percent of orders were redundant. EMR-S provide clinicians with a more current, comprehensive view of patient information—test results. EMR-S equipped with order entry and Clinical Decision Support features have the potential to reduce unnecessary tests by making physicians aware of current results and by alerting them to new orders that may be superfluous.

**Percentage Savings.** Three findings in the literature look at savings over a broad spectrum of laboratory tests, suggesting savings of 22.4 percent of the total outpatient laboratory costs. A number of findings for specific tests (urea, albumin, etc.) are also available. Because we know neither the distribution nor the base cost for those tests, we were unable to use them. The range of savings for those findings is 6 to 88 percent.

**Extrapolation of Savings.** We do not currently know what expenditures on laboratory tests are generated by the average physician. Wang et al. (2003) reported that physicians with capitated patients spend $27,600 each year on laboratory tests. This figure is based on Boston's Partners HealthCare System and might be high as a country average, leading to overestimating the laboratory savings for the outpatient sector.

Fortunately, this overestimate would be partially compensated for by an underestimate of the laboratory savings in the inpatient setting. The reason is that we use the outpatient national base cost to estimate the inpatient national base cost, which is obtained by subtracting the outpatient national base cost from the total (outpatient and inpatient) national base cost. Using the figure from Wang et al. (2003), we estimate that the national base cost (NBC) for outpatient laboratory test is $NBC_o = \$11.4$ billion. In a study of the diagnostics industry, Marketdata Enterprises (2002a, b) estimated the size of this market at $41.7 billion in 2001. Applying their estimated rate of growth, we calculated the size of the entire market in 2004 as NBC = $49.8 billion; therefore, the size of the market for the inpatient sector at $NBC_i = \$38.4$ billion. Let us, for simplicity, assume that the delay $\tau$ is the same in the inpatient and outpatient sectors and let us denote by $PS^{Lab}$ the aggregate potential savings (PS) from reduced laboratory tests, in both the inpatient and outpatient sectors. Then, the elasticity[1] of the laboratory potential savings ($PS^{Lab}$) with respect to the outpatient national base cost ($NBC_o$) is

$$\frac{\partial PS^{Lab}}{\partial NBC_o} \frac{NBC_o}{PS^{Lab}} = \frac{1}{1 + \dfrac{s_o NBC}{(s_o - s_i)NBC_o}} \approx 0.17, \tag{3.1}$$

where $s_o$ and $s_i$ are the percentage savings in the outpatient sector and inpatient sector, respectively. This implies that even if the outpatient national base cost $B_o$ is overestimated by 30 percent, the *total* laboratory potential savings ($PS^{Lab}$) are overestimated by 5 percent. Since the laboratory potential savings are small with respect to the aggregate national potential savings, this error would create a minuscule overestimate of the aggregate potential savings of 0.3 percent. This small overestimate suggests that, although we report the figures for the laboratory savings separately for the inpatient and outpatient sectors, the most reliable figure is their sum.

**National Savings.** From the figures reported above, we estimated that the potential savings from reduction in laboratory tests are $2.2 billion, corresponding to mean yearly savings of $1.1 billion and cumulative savings over 15 years of $15.9 billion.

---

[1] The *elasticity* of quantity $y$ with respect to quantity $x$ is $\Delta y/\Delta x \times x/y$ and can be used to quantify the percentage change in $y$ associated with a percentage change in $x$.

**Drug Utilization**

Computerized Physician Order Entry (CPOE) and Clinical Decision Support (CDS) features of EMR-S can potentially lower drug costs by structuring medication selections to align with formulary rules; advising physicians of the cost-benefit characteristics of specific drugs at the time of ordering; recommending less-expensive alternative drugs, including generics; encouraging providers to discontinue unneeded or contraindicated medications; and encouraging timely conversion from intravenous to oral medications.

The computation of the savings due to reduced drug utilization is more complicated than the previous ones. It combines the following three styles of calculations:

- Wang et al. (2003) report that HIT could lead to a 15-percent reduction in drug utilization. The authors argue that these savings apply only to capitated patients. However, it is difficult to imagine that once an EMR-S is in place, only some patients would benefit from it. Therefore, we apply a flat 15-percent savings in outpatient drug expenditures. Heffler et al. (2004) report U.S. expenditures in 2002 for retail prescription drugs at $162.4 billion, and they project them at $207.9 billion for 2004, a figure that includes both inpatient and outpatient sectors. To separate the two, we rely on a report by Johnston et al. at the Center for Information Technology Leadership (CITL) (2003), which sets the outpatient component at 77 percent of the total. This suggests that the national-level base cost is $160 billion, which implies a potential savings of $20.4 billion. If we did not take into account the 15 percent of physicians who have adopted already, the savings would be $24 billion, a figure quite close to the $27 billion estimated by CITL (Johnston et al., 2003).
- One report by Cap Gemini Ernst & Young (2000) claims that there is a potential savings of $0.75–$3.2 per prescription. The National Association of Chain Drug Stores reports 3.14 billion scripts in 2002. From Heffler et al. (2004), which quotes figures from the CMS National Health Expenditures (NHE), we find U.S. expenditures in 2002 for retail prescription drugs of $162.4 billion. Therefore, the average expenditure per script is $51.8, which is in excellent agreement with data reported by the Kaiser Family Foundation (http://www.statehealthfacts.kff.org/), which is $52.97 (inflation should be taken into account). Therefore, the Cap Gemini Ernst & Young study suggests that one could achieve savings in the $2.3- to $10-billion range. Applying the growth rate in drug expenditures estimated by Heffler et al. (2004), we see this range inflated to $3 billion–$12.9 billion, with an average of $7.9 billion. Once we take into account a current adoption rate of 15 percent, we obtain a range of potential savings of $2.6 billion–$11 billion, with an average of $6.7 billion.
- In another study, Cap Gemini Ernst & Young (2004) looked at a clinic with five physicians and documented savings per physician in the $13,400–$19,000

range. Since the study was done in 1998, we adjusted the values according to the growth in drug expenditures (138 percent), obtaining a savings of $38,556 per physician and a potential national savings of $13.5 billion.

**National Savings.** Using the figures reported above, we estimated that the potential savings from reduction in drug utilization are $12.9 billion, corresponding to mean yearly savings of $6.2 billion and cumulative savings over 15 years of $92.3 billion.

### Radiology/Imaging

**Percentage Savings.** To date, we have only one estimate of savings in outpatient radiology expenditures: The paper by Wang et al. (2003) reports savings of 14 percent, based on the consensus of a panel of experts.

**Extrapolation of Savings.** The amount spent at the national level on radiology and imaging is not well estimated. CITL (Johnston et al., 2003) estimates that the United States spends $64 billion a year on radiology. A document of the Atlantic Imaging Group (2005) sets this number at $46 billion, whereas a document from National Imaging Associates (2000) sets it at $75 billion in 1998. The most thorough source found so far is Sunshine, Mabry, and Bansal (1991), which sets this number in the $19–$22 billion range in 1990. The real yearly growth rate of health spending has been around 5 percent in the past decade. Since it is known that radiology expenditures grew faster than the average, we use a rate of 6 percent, which leads to a national-level estimate of $40.5 billion–$47 billion in 2004. Averaging all these estimates, we obtained a base cost of $56.4 billion.

This estimate includes inpatient and outpatient costs. To get the outpatient portion, we deducted the amount for the inpatient costs, 4 percent of total expenditures in 2001, which we obtained from the Healthcare Cost Report Information System (HCRIS) dataset (Centers for Medicare & Medicaid Services, 2005b). Since projected hospital expenditures for 2004 are $551.7 billion, we estimated inpatient radiology expenditures in 2004 at $22 billion. This leads to an outpatient level of expenditures on radiology of $34.4 billion.

In Wang et al. (2003) the radiology expenditures per physician are set at $59,100, which implies a national-level base cost of $24.4 billion. Taking the average of our two estimates, we obtained national-level outpatient radiology expenditures equal to $29.4 billion.

**National Savings.** From the figures reported above, we estimated the potential savings from a reduction in radiology expenditures to be $3.6 billion, corresponding to mean yearly savings of $1.7 billion and cumulative savings over 15 years of $25.6 billion.

## Inpatient

Hospital care accounts for about one-third of national health expenditures (which were $1,679 billion in 2003). Therefore, even modest percentage savings brought about by HIT in the inpatient setting have the potential to save large amounts of money. The inpatient setting shares some features with the ambulatory setting that allow EMR-S to bring similar types of savings. In particular, we documented inpatient savings related to reductions in laboratory tests, drug utilization, and handling of medical records. While there is evidence that Picture Archiving and Communications Systems are associated with considerable savings, the literature findings on PACS were not easily scalable at the national level, and so we omitted them at this stage. Most of the savings in the inpatient setting seem to be realized when HIT enables a transformation of the process of care, as documented by findings related to reductions in length of stay and nurses' unproductive time. We detail our findings in the following five subsections.

### Reduction of Nurses' Unproductive Time

Nursing Documentation Systems, which allow nurses to assess patients, document care, and, in some cases, enter orders online at the patient's bedside, yield savings by reducing the time nurses spend on documentation, redundant data collection, and patient assessment; the ratio of high- to less-skilled positions; and the costs associated with paper forms; and preventing many missed charges. Decision rules in such systems can coordinate care by automatically alerting ancillary services, such as dietary or social workers, through the documented entries. In this analysis, we focus on reductions in documentation time. The time saved on documentation could be used in at least three ways: (1) to reduce the number of employed nurses; (2) to take better care of the same number of patients; and (3) to take care of additional patients, keeping quality constant. In this document we consider the third scenario, based on the fact that there appears to be reasonable consensus that there is a shortage of nurses that is projected to continue for several years ahead (Bureau of Health Professions, 2002; Spetz and Given, 2003; HSM Group Ltd., 2002; Buerhaus, Staiger, and Auerbach, 2000, 2003). Therefore we make the assumption that a reduction in nurses' unproductive time will translate into a reduction of the demand for nurses.

**Percentage Savings.** The direct evidence about the size of the effect of HIT on reduction of nurses' unproductive time consists of the following three findings. These findings differ in reliability and generalizability; therefore, we felt that it was important to assign to them a set of subjective weights, to prevent possible overestimation.

- A study of nurses in intensive care units (ICUs) (Wong et al., 2003) reports that the percentage of time spent on documentation decreased by 52 minutes per each 8-hour shift, allowing nurses to spend more time with patients. Keeping the nurse-to-patient ratio fixed, this translates into an 11-percent reduction in the demand for nurses. We assign to this finding a weight of 1.
- A report on EMR-S in Norwegian hospitals (Ellingsen and Monteiro, 2003) quotes a 10-percent savings in nurses' time. We assign to this finding a weight of 0.5, since it applies to a foreign country with a very different health care system. In addition, although the quote appears in a peer-reviewed article, the original source for this number is not available.
- In Fickel (2001), published on Oracle's website (www.oracle.com/oramag/profit/01-Nov/p41industry.html), the author quotes savings in nurses' time of between 12 and 20 percent. These numbers, however, appear to be vendors' estimates of what may happen. We assign to this finding a weight of 0.25: Although it seems worthwhile to report it, we are not sure how reliable this finding is, and we do not want it to have much influence on our estimates.

These findings suggest that HIT could lead to a reduced demand for nurses of 11.4 percent, a value that is consistent with conversations we had with hospital executives and nurses during site visits to hospitals.

**Extrapolation of Savings: A Lower Bound.** The model for the computation of savings is slightly different from what we presented in Chapter Two. We consider the case of no delay ($\tau=1$) just for notational simplicity, although we did include the delay in the actual computations. Let $D_t$ be the demand for nurses in year $t$, and let $w_t$ be the yearly wages of nurses. In this context, we use the word *demand* (*supply*) to mean "quantity demanded" ("supplied"). Since the market is in disequilibrium now, with demand exceeding supply, it is reasonable to expect that wages will rise over time until the market clears, so that $w_t > w_{2004}$. The expenditures on nurses in year $t$ are given by $E_t = w_t D_t$. Let us now consider a scenario in which we introduce HIT innovations that reduce the demand for nurses to $D_t^* < D_t$. This reduction in demand will be paralleled by a reduction in wages, which we now denote by $w_t^* < w_t$. Expenditures on nurses under this scenario will be $E_t^* = w_t^* D_t^*$. Yearly savings to *all* providers will then be $S_t = E_t - E_t^* = w_t D_t - w_t^* D_t^*$. If the innovation in HIT is adopted according to the adoption curve $p_t$, the demand for nurses $D_t^*$ will be $D_t - sD_t p_t$, so that savings are

$$ S_t = s w_t^* p_t D_t + D_t \left( w_t - w_t^* \right). \tag{3.2} $$

Therefore, savings accrue both because the number of nurses hired is lower than expected and because the reduced demand leads to lower wages ($w_t^* < w_t$). Although, in principle, it would be possible to estimate both $w_t$ and $w_t^*$, using an approach similar to the one described in Spetz and Given (2003), the estimation of the term $w_t - w_t^*$ is beyond the scope of this project. We settle for a lower bound on the savings by setting $w_t = w_t^* = w_{2004}$—that is, by neglecting the savings due to the decrease in wages. Subtracting the savings that accrue to providers who have already adopted in year 2004, we obtain a final expression for yearly savings:

$$S_t = s w_{2004} D_t \left( p_t - p_{2004} \right). \tag{3.3}$$

We have already estimated that $s=0.114$, so we need $w_{2004}$ and $D_t$ to compute national savings figures. We estimated the yearly wage by taking the point of view of the employer. The National Compensation Survey of the Bureau of Labor Statistics (http://www.bls.gov/ncs/home.htm) sets the average hourly cost of registered nurses to employers at $37.23 ($26.53 is wages and salary, and the rest is benefits), and we use an average of 2,000 hours worked per year, which corresponds to 40 hours/week for 50 weeks.

The predicted demand for nurses is taken from work by the Bureau of Health Professions (BHP, 2002), an agency belonging to the Department of Health and Human Services. The BHP took into account factors such as the increase in population, a larger proportion of elderly persons, and medical advances that heighten the need for nurses and produced a forecast of the demand for nurses until the year 2020. The demand for nurses produced by BHP and the demand for nurses $D_t^*$ under the scenario of HIT adoption are shown in Figure 3.1.

**How Low Is the Lower Bound?** It is important to have an idea of what the size of the term we neglect in Equation (3.2) might be. To this end, we perform a simple comparative static exercise and assume that the labor market is in equilibrium. Dropping the time subscript $t$, since it is not used, let the labor supply be denoted by $L(w)$ and let us assume that it has constant elasticity $\alpha$, so that $L(w) \propto w^\alpha$. Let us explicitly model demand as a function of the percentage savings $s$ and write $D(s) \equiv D(0) - spD(0)$, where $p$ is the adoption rate. In equilibrium, quantity supplied and quantity demanded are equal, implying that $w(s) \propto D(s)^{1/\alpha}$. Therefore, expenditures on nurses are $E(s) \propto D^{1+1/\alpha} s$. A simple computation shows that the percentage reduction in expenditures due to HIT is

$$\frac{E(0) - E(s)}{E(0)} = 1 - (1 - ps)^{1 + \frac{1}{a}} \approx (1 + \frac{1}{a}) ps, \tag{3.4}$$

where the approximation holds if $ps \ll 1$. The expression above shows that the savings due to reduced wages are inversely proportional to the supply elasticity of labor, and

**Figure 3.1**
**BHP-Projected Demand for Nurses ($D_t$) (Bureau of Health Professions, 2002) and the Demand for Nurses Under a HIT-Adoption Scenario ($D_t'$)**

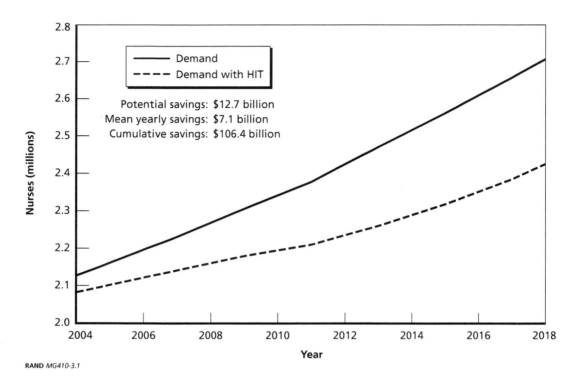

RAND MG410-3.1

they are $1/\alpha$ the savings due to reduced nursing hours. Our lower bound corresponds to the assumption that labor is perfectly elastic, so that $\alpha=\infty$. If the elasticity of labor supply were equal to 1, then the term we neglect would have the same size as the term we include, and an elasticity lower than 1 would make it larger.

**National Savings.** From the figures reported above, we estimated that the potential savings from a reduction in nurses' unproductive time are $12.7 billion, corresponding to mean yearly savings of $7.1 billion and cumulative savings over 15 years of $106.4 billion.

## Laboratory Tests

EMR-S have the potential to reduce test utilization by providing clinicians convenient views of current results, thus reducing orders for redundant lab tests or images. Clinical Decision Support rules can alert clinicians to unnecessary tests (as well as reminding them of needed tests based on current medications or changes in a patient's condition). Structured order sets can help standardize test ordering and further reduce redundancy.

**Percentage Savings.** In Tierney and Miller (1993), laboratory charges were shown to be reduced by 12.5 percent. In Wu, Peters, and Morgan (2002), results from a Toronto hospital show a reduction in total number of tests by 11 percent. Therefore, we use an average of 11.8 percent savings in laboratory costs.

The Tierney and Miller study dates back to 1993, and it relates the results of the Regenstrief Medical Record System, which was one the nation's first EMR-S. One could object that this evidence is old and may no longer apply, and also that it may represent a best-case scenario. This study is used to provide three out of the 10 findings for savings in the inpatient setting: reduction in length of stay (10.5 percent), laboratory tests (12.5 percent), and drug utilization (15.2 percent); therefore, it is reasonable to ask how much our results depend on this particular piece of evidence. If we set the percentage savings from this reference to half of their values, our inpatient potential savings drop by 12 percent. However, while there are reasons that many hospitals may not achieve the savings reported by Tierney and Miller, there are also reasons for hospitals achieving larger savings. For example, because the finding is 10 years old, and EMR-S have improved a great deal since 1993, we would expect better performance now than then. We note that our estimates of savings are quite small, somewhere between 10 and 15 percent, which leaves ample space for improvement. In addition, while relative to 1993, the Regenstrief experience is a best-case scenario, it is not immediately obvious that it is a best-case scenario for 2004, by which so much more experience on the implementation of EMR-S has been gained. Our main point is that both smaller and larger savings might be realized, and we take this fact into account by attaching a large standard deviation to our estimates, as we discuss in the "Quantifying Uncertainty in Savings Estimates" subsection.

**Extrapolation of Savings.** In a study of the laboratory diagnostic testing industry, Marketdata Enterprises estimated the size of this market at $41.7 billion in 2001. Applying their estimated rate of growth, we obtained a size of the market in 2004 of $49.8 billion. As explained in more detail in the "Quantifying Uncertainty in Savings Estimates" subsection, we estimated the outpatient portion of this market at one-fifth, which implies that hospitals spend about $39.8 billion a year on laboratory tests. We validated this result against an alternative form of calculations. Kane and Siegrist (2002) studied a large number of acute hospitals and found that the laboratory cost center is responsible for about 8 percent of the total cost. Applying this percentage to the projected $551.7 billion of hospital expenditures reported in Heffler et al. (2004), we estimated that in 2004 hospitals spent $44.1 billion on laboratory tests. Since it is likely that laboratory expenditures for non–acute care hospitals are lower, the $44.1-billion figure may provide an upper bound for laboratory expenditures at the national level, in good agreement with the $39.8 billion estimated above.

**National Savings.** On the basis of the figures reported above, we estimated that the potential savings from a reduction in laboratory tests are $3 billion, corresponding to mean yearly savings of $1.6 billion and cumulative savings over 15 years of $23.4 billion.

## Drug Utilization

**Percentage Savings.** The most solid piece of evidence showing savings in drug utilization in the inpatient setting is described in Tierney and Miller (1993), in which the authors performed a randomized clinical trial and found a reduction of 15.2 percent in drug costs.

**Extrapolation of Savings.** Using the Medicare Market Basket projections (Centers for Medicare & Medicaid Services, 2005c) for the year 2004, we estimated that hospital expenditures on pharmaceuticals are 7.3 percent of the total hospital expenditures, or $40.3 billion. To validate this result, we looked at a report by Kane and Siegrist (2002), who found that pharmaceuticals account for 7.9 percent of the total costs of acute hospitals. Our national-level base cost estimate of $40.3 billion is also in excellent agreement with the figure of $37.9 billion quoted by Health Strategies Group's study of hospital pharmacy trends (2004).

## Reduction in Length of Stay

Patient flow through the inpatient setting is subject to a multitude of delays—for example, delays in the ordering process, including waiting for written orders to be transcribed and communicated; delays caused by errors, as when a needed test is inadvertently ordered late; delays in task prioritization; delays in ordering ancillary services following nursing assessment, in searching for paper documents before visiting a patient, and in coordinating all of the information and communications necessary for discharge planning. Such delays can be ameliorated by an EMR-S. CPOE systems such as the one described in Tierney and Miller (1993) can improve the problems piecemeal; eventually, integrated clinical information systems equipped with standardized care plans such as the one implemented at Ohio State University Medical Center or Maimonides Medical Center promise to have a larger impact on inpatient length of stay (LOS).

**Percentage Savings.** There is a wide range of estimates on reduction in length of stay. Tierney and Miller (1993) find an LOS reduction of 10.5 percent in a randomized control trial. Mekhjian et al. (2002) find a statistically significant 5.1-percent reduction in the Ohio State University Hospitals, although they do not find a significant reduction at a cancer hospital. The lack of an effect at the cancer hospital is not too surprising, given the patients' conditions, and should be, in principle, taken into account when performing the aggregation at the national level. However, since there are relatively few cancer hospitals in the United States, we do not make this correction, which would be very insignificant. The Davies Award–winning Maimonides Medical Center in New York reported a 30-percent reduction in LOS (Baldwin, 2003), from 7.26 to 5.05 days. The average of these numbers gives a reduction in LOS of 15.2 percent.

**Extrapolation of Savings.** We present first our original calculation for the LOS-related savings, the one that is reported in Hillestad et al. (2005). We recently came across new data that allow us to derive a more reliable and principled estimate. The derivation of this new estimate, which is extremely close to our original one, is presented afterward.

To convert a reduction in length of stay to a dollar amount, we need to make assumptions on how HIT affects the LOS. We denote by $c(t)$ the cost per unit of time of an admission in a hospital without an EMR-S, and by $T$ the LOS for this admission. The cost of such an admission is

$$C \equiv \int_0^T c(\tau)d\tau. \tag{3.5}$$

Because HIT brings a change in the entire process of care, we model its effect on the cost per unit of time as a "time contraction": Procedures that used to be performed at time $t$ are performed, using HIT, at an earlier time, which is a fraction $(1-s)t$ of the original time. Therefore, denoting by $c^{HIT}(t)$ the cost of unit of time in a hospital with an EMR-S, we set

$$c^{HIT}([1-s]t) \equiv c(t) \Rightarrow c^{HIT}(t) \equiv c\left(\frac{t}{1-s}\right). \tag{3.6}$$

Therefore, the cost of the admission using HIT is

$$C^{HIT} = \int_0^{(1-s)T} c^{HIT}(\tau)d\tau = \int_0^{(1-s)T} c\left(\frac{\tau}{1-s}\right)d\tau = (1-s)C. \tag{3.7}$$

This reasoning suggests that, when we convert a reduction in LOS to a dollar figure, we should use the average cost of hospital days, rather than the marginal cost (that is, the cost of an additional day), because the HIT intervention is extended through the entire stay.

Given this assumption, there are at least two ways to estimate the base cost for the savings coming from a reduction in LOS:

- One could argue that, in the long run, a percentage reduction in LOS is matched by an equal percentage reduction in hospital operating expenditures. To get operating expenses from the National Health Expenditure figure of $551.7 billion, we computed total cost by assuming an average margin of 4.6 percent (American Hospital Association, 2002) and then subtracted new and old capital expenditures, which we estimated at 8 percent of total cost using the HCRIS datasets, obtaining a value of $477 billion.

- One could argue that only inpatient hospital expenditures should be taken into account. Since the ratio of inpatient expenditures to total expenditures is about 60 percent (http://www.cms.hhs.gov/charts/series/sec1.ppt), the base cost would be $286.2 (allocating all the capital expenditures to the inpatient sector).

For our calculation, we took as the base cost the average of the numbers estimated by each method, which is $387.4 billion.

**National Savings.** Using the figures reported above, we estimated that the potential savings from reduction in length of stay are $36.7 billion, corresponding to mean yearly savings of $19.3 billion and cumulative savings over 15 years of $289.6 billion.

**An Alternative, More Reliable Estimate.** As this report was about to be printed, we came across a study published in 2002 by K. Carey, an economist at the U.S. Department of Veterans Affairs who has studied hospital costs at length. This study analyzes total billed patient charges in about 20 percent of U.S. hospitals and finds an elasticity of 0.7 with respect to length of stay, arguing that hospitals save significant amounts of money by reducing length of stay. Since billed charges are proportional to expenditures, the elasticity figures can be applied to national hospital non-capital expenditures. If we use this value for our computations, we obtain a potential savings of $34.4 billion, instead of the $36.7 billion we reported in Hillestad et al. (2005). This estimate will be included in future versions of one of the author's (FG's) work. Carey recognizes that there could be still some upward omitted variable bias in her estimates, but even dropping the elasticity by 25 percent, from 0.7 to 0.525 we obtain a savings of $25.8 billion, which is still very sizable and would not alter our conclusions.

## Medical Records

As in the outpatient sector, HIT could bring savings in the medical records department and in all activities that require chart pulls.

**Percentage Savings.** We have not found evidence in the literature of savings of this type. However, we have gathered information from hospital executives and have concluded that it is plausible that medical records expenditures may be reduced by 50 percent.

**Extrapolation of Savings.** From our analysis of the HCRIS dataset, we estimated that 1.5 percent of total hospital expenditures is dedicated to medical records and medical record libraries. This estimate implies that the base cost for 2004 is $7.9 billion.

**National Savings.** Using the figures reported above, we estimated that the potential savings from a reduction in maintenance of medical records are $2.5 billion, corresponding to mean yearly savings of $1.3 billion and cumulative savings over 15 years of $19.9 billion.

## Summary of Savings at the National Level

In the preceding section, we quantified the savings for 10 savings categories. Here, we summarize the findings and aggregate the savings over the 10 categories. For each category of savings $i$ ($i=1, \ldots, 10$), the yearly savings $S_t^i$ can be written as

$$S_t^i\left(\tau_i\right) = \frac{s_i B_i N_i}{\tau_i} \sum_{k=1}^{\tau_i}\left(p_{t+k-1} - \hat{p}_{t+k-1}\right), \tag{3.8}$$

where $s_i$, $B_i$, and $N_i$ are, respectively, the percentage savings, the base cost, and the number of providers for category $i$ of savings, and $\tau_i$ is the implementation time, which is 2 years for the outpatient sector and 4 years for the inpatient sector. The product $s_i B_i N_i$ is related to the potential savings by Equation (2.12) and is reported for completeness in Table 3.1.

The aggregate national savings are simply computed as

$$S_t \equiv \sum_{i=1}^{10} S_t^i\left(\tau_i\right). \tag{3.9}$$

Expression (3.9) can now be used to compute savings at a fixed time in the future. For each savings category in Table 3.2, we report, for each savings category, the potential, mean yearly and cumulative savings, as well as the savings at year 5, 10 and 15 in the future (with the base year being 2004). We also report the aggregate savings over the outpatient setting, the inpatient setting, and the entire health sector.

**Table 3.1**
**The Product *sBN*, Necessary to Compute Yearly Savings, for Each Category of Savings**

| Savings Category | sBN ($billions) |
|---|---|
| Outpatient | |
| Transcription | 2.3 |
| Chart Pulls | 2.1 |
| Laboratory Tests | 2.7 |
| Drug Utilization | 15.9 |
| Radiology | 4.4 |
| Inpatient | |
| Nurse Shortage | 19.9 |
| Laboratory Tests | 4.7 |
| Drug Utilization | 5.8 |
| Length of Stay | 57.6 |
| Medical Records | 4 |

**Table 3.2**
**Summary of HIT-Enabled Efficiency Savings**

| Payers: Any | Potential Savings | Mean Yearly Savings | Cumulative Savings | Savings Year 5 | Savings Year 10 | Savings Year 15 |
|---|---|---|---|---|---|---|
| | | | ($billions) | | | |
| Outpatient | | | | | | |
| Transcription | 1.9 | 0.9 | 13.4 | 0.4 | 1.2 | 1.7 |
| Chart Pulls | 1.7 | 0.8 | 11.9 | 0.4 | 1.1 | 1.5 |
| Laboratory Tests | 2.2 | 1.1 | 15.9 | 0.5 | 1.5 | 2.0 |
| Drug Utilization | 12.9 | 6.2 | 92.3 | 3.0 | 8.6 | 11.8 |
| Radiology | 3.6 | 1.7 | 25.6 | 0.8 | 2.4 | 3.3 |
| Total | 22.3 | 10.6 | 159.0 | 5.2 | 14.8 | 20.4 |
| Inpatient | | | | | | |
| Nurse Shortage | 12.7 | 7.1 | 106.4 | 3.4 | 10.0 | 13.7 |
| Laboratory Tests | 3.0 | 1.6 | 23.4 | 0.8 | 2.2 | 2.8 |
| Drug Utilization | 3.7 | 2.0 | 29.3 | 1.0 | 2.8 | 3.5 |
| Length of Stay | 36.7 | 19.3 | 289.6 | 10.1 | 27.6 | 34.7 |
| Medical Records | 2.5 | 1.3 | 19.9 | 0.7 | 1.9 | 2.4 |
| Total | 58.6 | 31.2 | 468.5 | 16.1 | 44.5 | 57.1 |
| Total | 80.9 | 41.8 | 627.5 | 21.3 | 59.2 | 77.4 |

For the entire sector, the potential savings are $80.9 billion, corresponding to a mean yearly savings of $41.8 billion and a cumulative savings, over 15 years, of $627.5 billion.

Obviously, the savings accrue at different rates over time to different entities. One could argue that, in the long run, they will accrue to payers. Under this assumption, one way to allocate the savings to payers is by using as a basis for allocation their current level of expenditures as reported in the NHE (Centers for Medicare & Medicaid Services, 2005a). This is obviously an oversimplification of a difficult problem, but we report it here as one example of this procedure, just to give an idea of what the payer-specific savings might be. In Table 3.3, we show the savings that would accrue to Medicare under these assumptions. More examples can be found in the interactive spreadsheet savings_by_payer.xls, which allows users to choose from a list of payers (Medicare, Medicaid, Public, Federal, State and Local, Private Health Insurance, Out of Pocket, Any).

All the figures reported here are clearly subject to a fair degree of uncertainty, an issue we discuss in the following section.

**Table 3.3**
**HIT-Related Savings That Would Accrue to Medicare**

| Payers:<br>Medicare | Potential<br>Savings | Mean<br>Yearly<br>Savings | Cumulative<br>Savings | Savings<br>Year 5 | Savings<br>Year 10` | Savings<br>Year 15 |
|---|---|---|---|---|---|---|
| | | | ($billions) | | | |
| Outpatient | | | | | | |
| Transcription | 0.4 | 0.2 | 2.7 | 0.1 | 0.3 | 0.3 |
| Chart Pulls | 0.3 | 0.2 | 2.4 | 0.1 | 0.2 | 0.3 |
| Laboratory Tests | 0.5 | 0.2 | 3.2 | 0.1 | 0.3 | 0.4 |
| Drug Utilization | 2.6 | 1.2 | 18.7 | 0.6 | 1.7 | 2.4 |
| Radiology | 0.7 | 0.3 | 5.2 | 0.2 | 0.5 | 0.7 |
| Total | 4.5 | 2.2 | 32.3 | 1.1 | 3.0 | 4.1 |
| Inpatient | | | | | | |
| Nurse Shortage | 3.9 | 2.2 | 32.7 | 1.0 | 3.1 | 4.2 |
| Laboratory Tests | 0.9 | 0.5 | 7.2 | 0.3 | 0.7 | 0.9 |
| Drug Utilization | 1.1 | 0.6 | 9.0 | 0.3 | 0.9 | 1.1 |
| Length of Stay | 11.3 | 5.9 | 88.9 | 3.1 | 8.5 | 10.7 |
| Medical Records | 0.8 | 0.4 | 6.1 | 0.2 | 0.6 | 0.7 |
| Total | 18.0 | 9.6 | 143.8 | 4.9 | 13.7 | 17.5 |
| Total | 22.5 | 11.7 | 176.1 | 6.0 | 16.7 | 21.7 |

## Quantifying Uncertainty in Savings Estimates

The savings estimates shown in Tables 3.2 and 3.3 are uncertain for a variety of reasons. The major source of uncertainty is the key quantity that determines the potential savings: the product $s_i B_i N_i$, where $s_i$ is the percentage savings, $B_i$ is the base cost per provider, and $N_i$ is the total number of providers. However, there is also uncertainty in the parameters of the adoption curve, such as the adoption time $T_{10 \to 90}$ and the current adoption rate $p_{2004}$. Here, we wish to quantify how this uncertainty is reflected in the aggregate savings $S_t$ of Equation (3.9).

The standard way to measure the uncertainty in $S_t$ follows four steps: (1) Assign probability distributions to the product $s_i B_i N_i$ and to the parameters $T_{10 \to 90}$ and $p_{2004}$, (2) draw a large number of samples from these distributions, (3) plug these values into the definition of $S_t$, and (4) obtain, for each year $t$, a distribution of values $S_t$, which can then be plotted.

The main difficulty in this process is choosing a reasonable standard deviation for the product $s_i B_i N_i$, and in particular for the term $s_i$, which is the crucial parameter of the entire exercise. In fact, in most cases the literature findings on HIT effects are sparse and cannot be used to estimate the standard deviation for $s_i$. However, they can be used for savings in transcription and chart pulls, for which we have 11 and 12 observations, respectively. Therefore, our strategy for assigning a probability distribution to all the products $s_i B_i N_i$ is as follows:

- We analyze transcription and chart pulls in detail and compute the coefficient of variations[2] in these two cases.
- We use these two coefficients to define an average coefficient of variation, which is then assumed to hold for every savings category.
- We compute the standard deviation for the product $s_i B_i N_i$, $i=1, \ldots, 10$, by multiplying its mean (reported in Table 3.1) by the coefficient of variation.

**Uncertainty of $s_i B_i N_i$ for Transcription Costs and Chart Pulls.** The average percentage savings $s_i$ are 0.735 and 0.634 for transcription and chart pulls, respectively, with corresponding standard deviations of 0.3 and 0.26, as reported in the spreadsheet savings_outpatient.xls. Since these parameters must be strictly between 0 and 1, we modeled them as random variables with a beta distribution.

To this uncertainty, we need to add the uncertainty about the base cost $B_i$ and the number of providers $N_i$ (which is the same in both cases). The base cost is $7,094 for transcription and $7,345 for chart pulls, and we modeled it with a uniform distribution centered around the mean value, with excursions of ±$1,500. The number of providers is 442,104, which we modeled with a uniform distribution centered around the mean, with excursions of ±100,000. Using these distributions, we found that the product $s_i B_i N_i$ has a coefficient of variation of 0.45 for both transcription and chart pulls, which we round to 0.5 for simplicity.

**Analysis of Uncertainty for the Aggregate Savings.** We now make the assumption that the coefficient of variation we have derived for transcription and chart pulls holds across all categories. This means that the products $s_i B_i N_i$ are modeled as random variables whose mean is given in Table 3.2 and whose standard deviation is simply half the mean. Since these variables are always positive, we model them with a gamma distribution, rather than normal distributions.

The only parameters left to model are those of the adoption curve. The adoption time is modeled with a gamma distribution with mean equal to 15 years and a standard deviation of 2 years, which basically implies variations between 10 and 20 years. The current adoption rate is modeled with a gamma distribution with means of 0.15 and 0.2 for outpatient and inpatient settings, respectively, and standard deviation of 0.05.

Using the probability distributions described above, we drew random values for $s_i B_i N_i$, as well as for the adoption curve $p_t$, generating random values for the aggregate savings $S_t$ using Equation (3.9). We drew 10,000 of such samples for each year $t$. The resulting distribution of $S_t$ is shown in Figure 3.2. The horizontal bar in the middle of the rectangle shown for each year is the mean value of $S_t$; the top and bottom of

---

[2] The *coefficient of variation* is the ratio between the standard deviation and the mean.

**Figure 3.2**
**Yearly Aggregate National Efficiency Savings and Their Uncertainty**

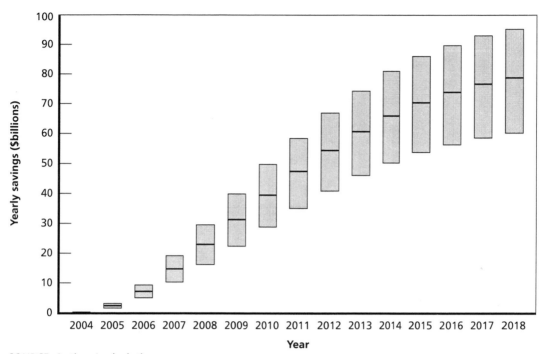

SOURCE: Authors' calculations.
NOTE: The horizontal bar in the middle of the rectangle shown for each year is the mean value; the top and bottom of the rectangle are the 80th and 20th percentiles, respectively.
RAND MG410-3.2

the rectangle are the 80th and 20th percentiles, respectively. Note that, as time progresses, the aggregate savings approach the potential savings of $80 billion reported in Table 3.2, and that the 20th and 80th percentiles are about $20 billion below and above the mean, respectively. It is important to note that we have modeled the random variables $s_i B_i N_i$ across savings categories as being independent, which might not be the case: Errors might be correlated across categories. Therefore, the assumption of independence should be seen as a simplifying assumption, which could lead to an underestimate of the standard deviation of the aggregate savings.

# CHAPTER FOUR

# Estimating the Cost of HIT

The savings described in the preceding chapter are contingent on the adoption of EMR-S in both inpatient and outpatient settings. In the following sections, we estimate how much it will cost providers to acquire and maintain these systems. We do not include in our calculations expenditures incurred to allow all the different components of the healthcare system to share patients' clinical information. Although such sharing is a very important component of HIT, none of the savings documented in the preceding chapter depends on such capabilities. A tentative estimate of the cost, but not the benefit, of "connecting" all the U.S. patients and providers is presented in Appendix C.

## Inpatient

To estimate the cost of placing an EMR-S in each U.S. hospital, we built a simple model of inpatient EMR-S costs, using data found in the literature or provided to us directly by hospitals, for a total of 27 hospitals. The model allows us to predict how much a hospital is likely to spend on an EMR-S, given basic hospital characteristics, such as size and operating expenses. The model does not tell us the specifics of the EMR-S, since our data are silent on these; rather it refers to a generic form of EMR-S, which includes elements of Computerized Physician Order Entry, patient records, and Picture Archiving and Communication Systems (PACS).

We divide the cost of EMR-S into two parts: a one-time, implementation cost and an annual operating, maintenance cost. The maintenance cost will be estimated as a percentage of the one-time cost, which is therefore the only one we need to model.

### One-Time Cost

The data are the 27 observations, one for each hospital. Each observation consists of the cost of an inpatient EMR-S, the number of beds covered by that EMR-S, the operating expenses of the hospital, and its teaching status. (It has been suggested that teaching hospitals might have different EMR-S costs from non-teaching hospitals.) The operating expenses and the number of beds refer to the last year of available data. Four data points come at an aggregate level, which means that the unit of observation is not a single hospital but a health system comprising a few hospitals that are treated as one large hospital. Of the 27 observations, 17 have been obtained directly from a large U.S. health system, which are, therefore, more reliable than the others, which have been obtained from the literature and from websites.

In most cases, the cost of the EMR-S is likely to be incurred over a period of three to five years. For the observations coming from the literature, we do not have a precise breakdown of the costs. For the observations coming from the health system, the cost includes hardware and software cost of the EMR-S itself, as well as local infrastructure expenses (such as wireless devices and desktop computers), and the labor costs of the hospital personnel involved in the implementation and in the redesign of hospital activities. The hardware costs also include costs associated with disaster-recovery hardware. A large component of the labor cost comes from training for the end users, and "leadership." Leadership costs include the expenses incurred in the process of obtaining the active participation and support of physicians and nurses.

A graph of the EMR-S cost as a function of both number of beds and operating expenses is shown in Figure 4.1. The data points labeled "Measured" correspond to the data given to us directly by a hospital system. The others ("Literature" and "Teaching") have either been found in the literature or been gathered informally from hospital executives. The data we used are available in the spreadsheet hospital_EMR-S_cost.xls.

Looking at Figure 4.1, we note that, except for the two large teaching hospitals, EMR-S costs are remarkably linear in operating expenses, suggesting that the process of EMR-S acquisition is budget-driven. Given our assumption that the EMR-S expenditure is incurred in a period of three to five years, our data imply that hospitals have spent from 1.8 to 3 percent of their operating expenses on the EMR-S acquisition. This number is in line with figures on IT spending often reported in the literature.

We can now build a simple model for the hospital expenditures on EMR-S. We denote by $C_i$ the cost of the EMR-S acquired by a hospital $i$ with $b_i$ beds, operating expenses $e_i$ and teaching status $t_i$ ($t_i$ is 1 for a teaching hospital and 0 otherwise). We model $C_i$ as a positive, random variable with the following distribution:

$$C_i \sim \Gamma(\mu(b_i, e_i, t_i; \boldsymbol{\theta}), \sigma^2), \qquad (4.1)$$

**Figure 4.1**
**Cost of Inpatient EMR-S as a Function of Beds and Operating Expenses**

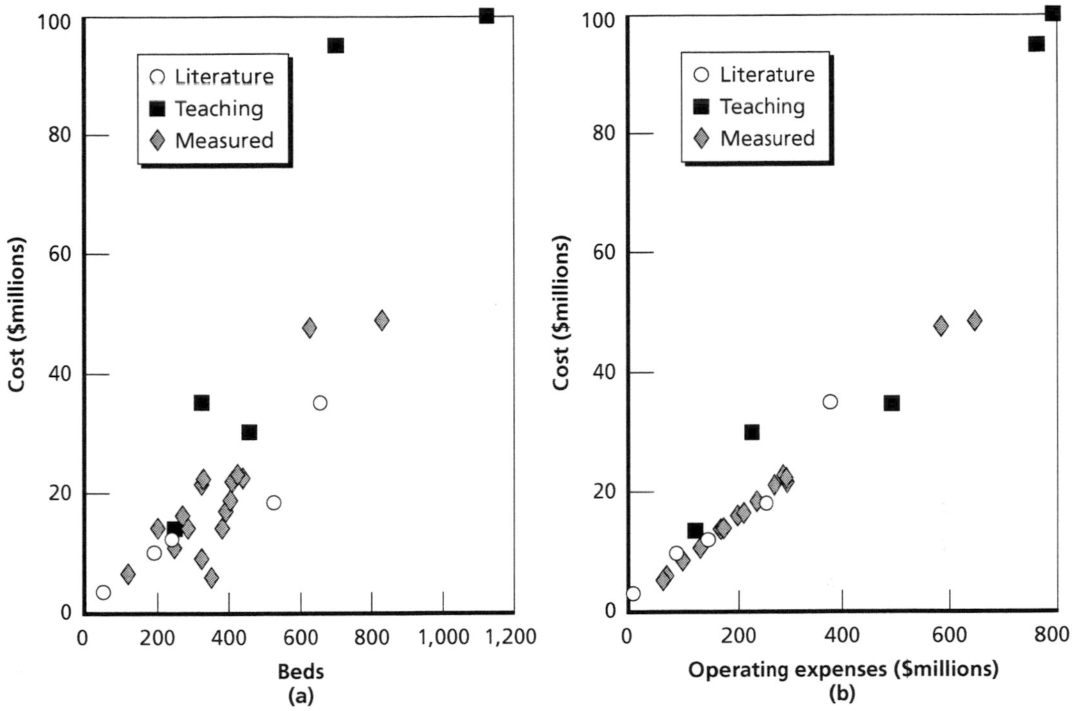

NOTE: See text for explanation. The data used to produce this figure can be found in the Excel spreadsheet hospital_EMR-S_cost.xls.

RAND *MG410-4.1*

where $\Gamma(\mu,\sigma^2)$ is the gamma density,[1] with mean $\mu$ and standard deviation $\sigma$. The mean of the gamma density is a function $\mu$ that depends on the covariates $b_i$, $e_i$, and $t_i$ through a specification with parameters $\theta$. We consider here the simplest specification for $\mu$:

$$\mu(b_i, e_i, t_i; \theta) \equiv \theta_0 + \theta_1 e_i + \theta_2 b_i + \theta_3 t_i. \qquad (4.2)$$

A variety of other specifications could be chosen (for example, Figure 4.1 suggests an interaction between teaching status and operating expenses). We did perform a more sophisticated analysis, reported in the following subsection, "Validation of the Regression Specifications," which takes into account the uncertainty on the specification $\mu$ and found that the simple linear specification (Equation [4.2]) well reproduces the results of that analysis, simply because of the strong linearity of the cost as a func-

---

[1] We use the gamma rather than the normal density because it is supported on the positive axis and will avoid generating negative costs.

tion of the operating expenses, which drives most of the result. The result of the estimation of Model (4.1) with Specification (4.2) is shown in Table 4.1.

Using the regression coefficients in Table 4.1, we can now predict the cost of an EMR-S for each U.S. hospital. To project the future cost of EMR-S acquisition by hospitals, we combined the standard, macro-level adoption theory with micro-simulations. The hospital data used in the microsimulation come primarily from the HCRIS dataset (Centers for Medicare & Medicaid Services, 2005b). The few data elements that were missing from HCRIS were derived from the American Hospital Association's yearly survey. We used the 2000 HCRIS, which at the time we began the study was the most complete of the datasets and was well linked to the AHA survey. The results were unchanged when we used the 2001 HCRIS. The HCRIS dataset includes all U.S. hospitals that take Medicare payments and, therefore, includes virtually all U.S. hospitals.

Our microsimulations proceeded as follows: We used the adoption curve described in Equation (2.3) to estimate the number of hospitals that will have an EMR-S in place in year $t$ (starting from the year 2004, for the next 15 years). Then, we randomly drew that number of hospitals from the hospitals represented in the HCRIS and computed their EMR-S cost using Specification (4.2). We assumed that it takes, on average, four years to complete the implementation; therefore, we spread the cost equally over the four years up to $t$. Maintenance costs are modeled as 30 percent of the one-time cost, or of the portion of the one-time cost incurred in the preceding year. The figure for the maintenance cost comes from conversations with one vendor and with the leaders of the implementation effort in one hospital system and in one large teaching hospital.

Using this process, we were able to estimate, for each year, how much hospitals will be spending on EMR-S. Consistent with our treatment of savings, we did not include in the total cost the expenditures of those hospitals that had started to implement an EMR-S during or before the year 2004. The resulting pattern of yearly expenditures is shown in Figure 4.2, where we also report the mean yearly cost (computed over 15 years) and the cumulative cost (also over 15 years). The

Table 4.1
Regression Estimates for Specification (4.2)

| | Estimate | Standard Error | t Value |
|---|---|---|---|
| Intercept | 1.9e+00 | 5.3e–01 | 3.7 |
| Operating Expense | 8.0e–02 | 6.7e–03 | 12.0 |
| Beds | –4.1e–03 | 4.0e–03 | –1.0 |
| Teaching | 7.4e+00 | 2.5e+00 | 2.9 |

**Figure 4.2**
**Yearly Expenditures on Inpatient EMR-S**

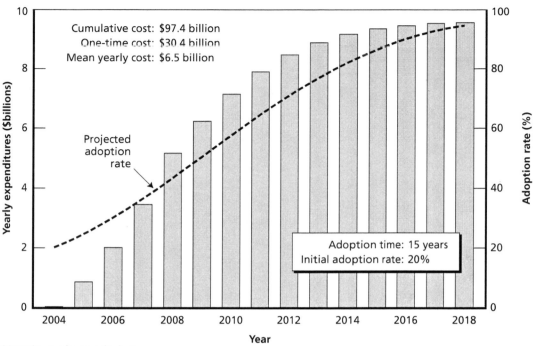

SOURCE: Authors' calculations.
RAND *MG410-4.2*

cumulative cost is split into a one-time cost component and a maintenance cost component. The one-time component is also reported in the figure.

Different results would be obtained by changing key adoption parameters, such as the adoption time or the initial adoption rate (here, set at 20 percent). In Table 4.2 we show how the cost figures change as a function of these two adoption parameters.

### Validation of the Regression Specifications

The cost estimates presented in this section have all been conditional on the choice of Specification (4.2), and one might be concerned that they are highly dependent on it. Here, we take a Bayesian approach and perform a slightly more complicated analysis, only to find that it is not worth the effort, since it leads to almost identical results.

Instead of considering just one specification, let us consider a series of $N$ plausible specifications $\mu_\gamma$, indexed by the integer index $\gamma$. Let us consider one measure of cost—say, the one-time cost—which is sufficient, because the other measures are

**Table 4.2**
**The Mean Yearly, One-Time, and Cumulative Costs of Inpatient**
**EMR-S for Different Choices of Adoption Parameters**

| | Adoption Time (years) | | |
|---|---|---|---|
| | 10 | 15 | 20 |
| Mean Yearly Cost ($billions) | | | |
| Initial adoption rate | | | |
| 0.15 | 7.6 | 6.8 | 5.6 |
| 0.20 | 6.7 | 6.5 | 5.6 |
| 0.25 | 5.9 | 6.0 | 5.4 |
| Cumulative Cost ($billions) | | | |
| Initial adoption rate | | | |
| 0.15 | 114.3 | 102.5 | 83.3 |
| 0.20 | 101.0 | 97.4 | 83.6 |
| 0.25 | 88.1 | 90.3 | 80.8 |
| One-Time Cost ($billions) | | | |
| Initial adoption rate | | | |
| 0.15 | 31.8 | 33.5 | 29.8 |
| 0.20 | 27.3 | 30.4 | 28.6 |
| 0.25 | 23.3 | 27.3 | 26.7 |

linearly related to it. To each specification $\mu_\gamma$, we can attach a one-time cost $C_\gamma$. Since there is uncertainty in the specification, we treat $\mu_\gamma$ as random variables, with probability density $P(\gamma)$ (which we leave unspecified for the moment), which implies that the one-time cost $C_\gamma$ is also a random variable with probability density $P(\gamma)$. Therefore, we can estimate the one-time cost by simply averaging over the specifications:

$$\bar{C} = \sum_{\gamma=1}^{N} C_\gamma P(\gamma) \tag{4.3}$$

The approach of the preceding section is equivalent to having a probability density $P(\gamma)$ that assigns probability 1 to Specification (4.2). An alternative is to consider all the specifications equiprobable and set $P(\gamma) = 1/N$. However, we are not indifferent to which specification we use, since some specifications may predict better than others; therefore, we proceed as follows. For each specification $\mu_\gamma$, we ran our regressions 1,000 times, each time leaving out four data points, which corresponds to about 15 percent of the data, and computing the absolute value of the prediction error on the four points left out. Denoting the average of these values by $\varepsilon_\gamma$, we simply set $P(\gamma) \propto 1/\varepsilon_\gamma^2$, assigning higher probability to those specifications that predict better the out-of-sample data.

We considered 12 different specifications. They include the basic linear specification with number of beds, operating expenses, and teaching status; a specification with operating expenses and all the possible interaction terms; and the basic linear specification with all the possible interaction terms:

$$\mu(b_i, e_i, t_i; \theta) \equiv \theta_0 + \theta_1 e_i + \theta_2 b_i + \theta_3 t_i$$

$$\mu(b_i, e_i, t_i; \theta) \equiv \theta_0 + \theta_1 e_i + \theta_2 e_i \times t_i$$

$$\mu(b_i, e_i, t_i; \theta) \equiv \theta_0 + \theta_1 e_i + \theta_2 e_i \times b_i$$

$$\mu(b_i, e_i, t_i; \theta) \equiv \theta_0 + \theta_1 e_i + \theta_2 b_i \times t_i$$

$$\mu(b_i, e_i, t_i; \theta) \equiv \theta_0 + \theta_1 e_i + \theta_2 b_i^2$$

$$\mu(b_i, e_i, t_i; \theta) \equiv \theta_0 + \theta_1 e_i + \theta_2 e_i^2$$

$$\mu(b_i, e_i, t_i; \theta) \equiv \theta_0 + \theta_1 e_i + \theta_2 t_i \qquad (4.4)$$

$$\mu(b_i, e_i, t_i; \theta) \equiv \theta_0 + \theta_1 e_i + \theta_2 e_i \times t_i + \theta_3 b_i + \theta_4 t_i$$

$$\mu(b_i, e_i, t_i; \theta) \equiv \theta_0 + \theta_1 e_i + \theta_2 e_i \times b_i + \theta_3 b_i + \theta_4 t_i$$

$$\mu(b_i, e_i, t_i; \theta) \equiv \theta_0 + \theta_1 e_i + \theta_2 b_i \times t_i + \theta_3 b_i + \theta_4 t_i$$

$$\mu(b_i, e_i, t_i; \theta) \equiv \theta_0 + \theta_1 e_i + \theta_2 b_i^2 + \theta_3 b_i + \theta_4 t_i$$

$$\mu(b_i, e_i, t_i; \theta) \equiv \theta_0 + \theta_1 e_i + \theta_2 e_i^2 + \theta_3 b_i + \theta_4 t_i$$

When we used the process outlined above with these 12 specifications, it turned out that the distribution of the one-time cost is very concentrated around the mean, with a coefficient of variation of 6 percent. In other words, the different specifications tend to provide the same result. In addition, the mean cost computed using this process is only 3 percent lower than the mean cost computed using the simple Specification (4.2), and therefore not significantly different from it, suggesting that there is no harm in using results obtained with that specification and making our calculations easier. If we had to use the method outlined above, each computation of cost would have to be repeated 12 times and then averaged using the weights $P(\gamma)$, creating an unnecessary computational burden.

## Outpatient

In this section, we describe physician expenditures on ambulatory EMR-S and project those expenditures into the future in order to obtain an estimate of the national cost of having an EMR-S in every physicians' office.

Our unit of observation is the physician practice (solo, dual, or group), and our model for the practice's expenditures is very simple: When a physician practice acquires an EMR-S, it incurs a fixed, one-time cost (cost of equipment plus setup cost); then, every year after that, it incurs a maintenance cost. We assumed that physicians acquire EMR-S according to the adoption curve described in Equation (2.3).

Next, we needed to document the cost of ambulatory EMR-S. There is no clear definition of an ambulatory EMR-S; therefore, we took a very inclusive view. To the best of our knowledge, the most complete information about cost of ambulatory EMR-S is available from Kirk Voelker, MD, and made publicly available at http://www.elmr-electronic-medical-records-emr.com/. The spreadsheet that documents both the cost and the features of more than 80 EMR-S products can be found at http://www.emrupdate.com/resources/downloads.aspx

For every product, the spreadsheet reports the acquisition cost (cost for one physician, three office staff), as well as the setup and annual maintenance costs. For our purposes, we simply take the sum of acquisition and setup costs to define the one-time cost, which covers both hardware and software costs. Maintenance cost includes the cost of software upgrades, license renewal, if necessary, and hardware upgrades (such as new monitors). For each product, the spreadsheet also reports up to 23 different features (such as "Prescriptions," "Practice Guidelines," "Billing Module," and "Reminders") and the number of users estimated by the vendor. We do not make use of that information here. Some of the products included in this spreadsheet have very low cost. Since the capabilities of those products are likely to be limited, we excluded such products, and any entry below $5,000 has been deleted from the data. Data from this spreadsheet have been augmented with data found in the white paper "Extensive Evaluation Ranks Top Electronic Medical Record Applications" by Anderson (2004).

As a result, we ended up with a table with 82 entries for the one-time cost. To each of these entries we added $3,000 to include additional hardware costs (such as printers) and a productivity loss of 15 percent for three months (based on an average yearly revenue of $150,000). The productivity loss takes into account the fact that it takes time, both for the physician and for the office staff, to learn to use the system, and that operation of the physician's practice is disrupted during the implementation time.

The final average cost of ambulatory EMR-S per physician turns out to be about $22,000, with a standard deviation of $6,000. The maintenance cost has been set at 20 percent of the one-time cost and, therefore, is about $4,400 per year. This figure is higher than the figure computed from the spreadsheet, but more in line with figures cited in the literature and with what we heard from experts.

To project expenditures into the future, we proceeded as follows:

- We randomly generated a set of about 170,000 practices of different sizes, consistent with data from Kane (2004).
- We randomly assigned to each physician practice a cost using the cost spreadsheet described above. We scaled the cost for a practice linearly with the number of physicians. We did not attempt to factor in economies of scale, since the evidence on this subject is mixed. We note, however, that the distribution of practice size is dominated by small practices: Almost 60 percent of physicians work in practices with up to four physicians. Therefore, unless economies of scale set in already at a small size (five or so), taking economies of scale into account would not lower the total cost figures by a large amount. The distribution of the one-time costs per physician across the 170,000 practices is shown in Figure 4.3.
- We generated an adoption curve according to the model of Equation (2.3), so that for each year we obtained an estimate for the number of "new adopters."
- For each year, a number of practices equal to the number of new adopters was drawn at random. All the physicians in those practices incurred a one-time cost (acquisition and setup). Yearly maintenance costs were computed as 20 percent of the one-time cost. As with the inpatient costs, we spread the one-time cost over an implementation period $\tau$. While for the inpatient setting we chose $\tau=4$, for the ambulatory setting a value of $\tau=2$ seemed more appropriate.
- For each year, we computed the total amount of money spent on EMR-S that year, including the acquisition and setup costs of the new adopters and the maintenance fees of the practices that had already adopted. We refer to this quantity as the *yearly expenditure*.

Every time we ran through this procedure, we generated a pattern of yearly expenditures over time. The patterns differ slightly from each other because the assignment of the cost to the physician practices is random, as are the particular practices that adopt every year. We ran this procedure many times (usually, 100) and computed the average of the yearly expenditures. Because of the large number of practices, the variance due to this randomness is very, very small (less than 1 percent of the mean); therefore, we report only point estimates.

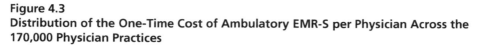

**Figure 4.3**
**Distribution of the One-Time Cost of Ambulatory EMR-S per Physician Across the 170,000 Physician Practices**

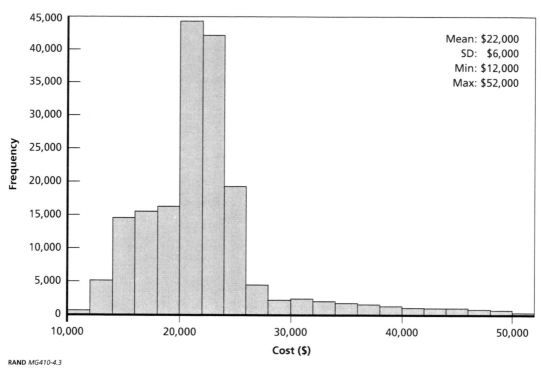

In Figure 4.4, we show the pattern of yearly expenditures computed using an adoption time of 15 years and an adoption rate in year 2004 of 15 percent. As with the inpatient costs, we do not include expenditures by physicians who decided to adopt in 2004. Note that we do not discount future cost, nor do we account for increases in the number of physicians or changes in costs.

The values varied as we varied key adoption parameters. In Table 4.3, we report the results of a sensitivity analysis over the adoption time and the initial adoption rate. The results are most sensitive to changes in adoption time. For example, by increasing the adoption time by one year, the mean yearly cost decreases by about 5 percent. Increasing the initial adoption rate by 1 percentage point leads to a decrease in mean yearly cost of only 1.5 percent.

**Figure 4.4**
**Yearly Expenditures on Ambulatory EMR-S**

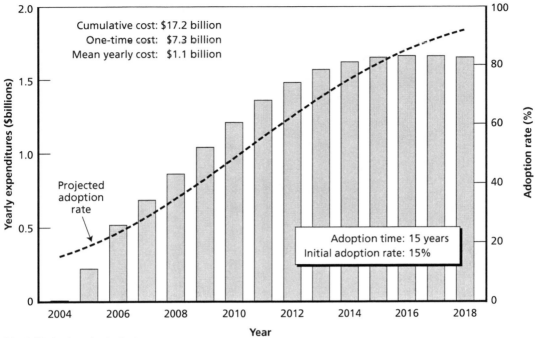

SOURCE: Authors' calculations.
**RAND** *MG410-4.4*

**Table 4.3**
**Cost of Ambulatory EMR-S for Different Values of Key Adoption Parameters**

|  | Adoption Time (years) | | |
| --- | --- | --- | --- |
|  | 10 | 15 | 20 |
| Mean Yearly Cost ($billions) | | | |
| Initial adoption rate | | | |
| 0.10 | 1.4 | 1.1 | 0.8 |
| 0.15 | 1.4 | 1.1 | 0.9 |
| 0.20 | 1.3 | 1.1 | 0.9 |
| Cumulative Cost ($billions) | | | |
| Initial adoption rate | | | |
| 0.10 | 21.2 | 16.3 | 12.0 |
| 0.15 | 20.9 | 17.2 | 13.5 |
| 0.20 | 20.0 | 17.1 | 14.1 |
| One-Time Cost ($billions) | | | |
| Initial adoption rate | | | |
| 0.10 | 8.3 | 7.4 | 5.8 |
| 0.15 | 7.7 | 7.3 | 6.1 |
| 0.20 | 7.1 | 6.9 | 6.1 |

# CHAPTER FIVE

# Simulation of Financial Incentives

The analysis of the preceding chapters suggests that large benefits are to be gained from HIT adoption and that the nation might benefit if the pace of HIT adoption were to quicken. In this chapter, we consider financial incentives aimed at increasing HIT-adoption rates. We will address the question of how much they could cost, whether the benefits would outweigh the costs, and how incentive parameters, such as size and duration, affect the benefit/cost ratio.

We do not have detailed data about how individual providers might react to financial incentives, so our modeling is very simple and is done at the aggregate level. In addition, to simplify the analysis, we assume here that the implementation phase is short, so that $\tau=1$. Since the value of $\tau$ affects only minimally ratios of savings and costs, and since we will be concerned with benefit/cost ratios, this simplification does not affect our conclusions.

To model incentives we need a simple extension of the adoption curve of Equation (2.3), in which we allow the diffusion speed $b$ to depend on time. Our adoption curve is now written as follows (with $m=1$):

$$p_{t+1} = p_t + D_t$$
$$D_t = b_t p_t (1 - p_t). \qquad (5.1)$$

The quantity $D_t=b_t p_t(1-p_t)$ is the number of providers that adopt during year $t$, and we interpret it as the demand for an EMR-S (where we have normalized the population of providers to 1). Here, year $t$ is defined as the time interval between $t$ and $t+1$, and $p_t$ is the number of providers who have an EMR-S at the beginning of year $t$. The interpretation of the demand term $D_t$ is very simple: This term comes from assuming that the probability that a provider who does not have an EMR-S in year $t$ will adopt one is proportional to the current adoption rate $p_t$, with a constant of proportionality equal to $b_t$. Therefore, the number of providers who will adopt an EMR-S in year $t$ is simply the probability $b_t p_t$ times the fraction of providers who do not have an EMR-S, given by $(1-p_t)$.

Since the demand for EMR-S must depend on the current price of EMR-S, the parameter $b_t$ must depend implicitly on the price of an EMR-S at time $t$, which we denote by $C_t$. It is important to note that the demand for EMR-S in year $t$ depends on the current price $C_t$ through the term $b$, and on the previous prices through the term $p_t$. Let us assume that the demand for EMR-S has constant price elasticity $\varepsilon$, so that

$$\frac{dD_t}{dC_t}\frac{C_t}{D_t} = -|\varepsilon|. \tag{5.2}$$

This elasticity measures the "instantaneous" responsiveness of the demand during year $t$ to a price change in year $t$, keeping everything else constant.

Substituting the definition of $D_t$ in this expression, and remembering that $b_t$ must be a function of $C_t$, we obtain a differential equation for $b_t$:

$$\frac{db_t}{dC_t}\frac{C_t}{b_t} = -|\varepsilon|, \tag{5.3}$$

whose solution is clearly

$$b_t = \frac{\alpha}{C_t^{|\varepsilon|}}, \tag{5.4}$$

where $\alpha$ is a numeric factor. This expression allows us to model the adoption process when the price of EMR-S changes over time. In fact, substituting Equation (5.4) into Equation (5.1), we obtain an adoption curve that follows the difference equation

$$p_{t+1} = p_t + \frac{\alpha}{C_t^{|\varepsilon|}} p_t (1 - p_t). \tag{5.5}$$

Let us assume that the market for EMR-S is currently in equilibrium, at price $C$, with a perfectly elastic supply, and that the current diffusion speed is $b$,[1] so that the parameter $\alpha$ is known from Equation (5.4).

We can now easily model a subsidy program: Assume that in year $t$ a percentage subsidy of size $X_t$ becomes available, reducing the cost of an EMR-S from $C$ to $C(1 - X_t)$. The adoption curve in the presence of such a subsidy will evolve as follows:

---

[1] Its value is about 0.3 (Bower, 2005), which corresponds to an adoption time of 15 years.

$$p_{t+1} = p_t + \frac{b}{(1-X_t)^{|\varepsilon|}}\, p_t(1-p_t). \qquad (5.6)$$

In this framework, the effect of a subsidy is simply to increase the adoption speed (the parameter $b$) in a time-dependent fashion. In most cases, we would expect a subsidy schedule of the form $(0,0, \ldots, X,X, \ldots, X,0,0, \ldots)$, which indicates that the subsidy program starts in a certain year, is available for a few years, and then stops. An example of the effect of a subsidy on the adoption curve is shown in Figure 5.1.

It is important to note that altering the price during year $t$ has two effects on the future adoption pattern: an instantaneous effect on demand during the same year, controlled by $\varepsilon$, and an "avalanche" effect, controlled by $b$, through the increased adoption rate in the next year, which, in turn, increases the adoption rate in the following year, and so on.

We used Equation (5.6) for two purposes: to estimate the value of a subsidy and to estimate the cost of a subsidy. The cost of the subsidy is easily estimated by using

**Figure 5.1**
**Adoption Curves With and Without a Subsidy**

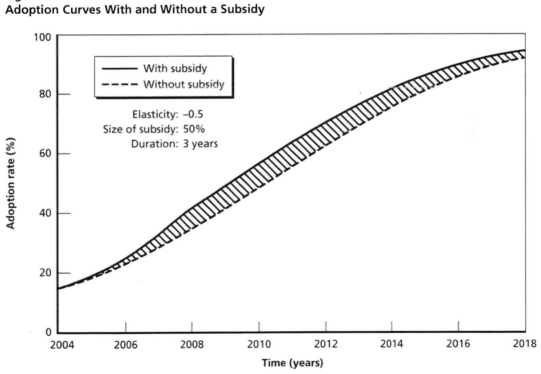

NOTE: In this figure, we consider a 50-percent subsidy that begins in the year 2006 and lasts three years, until 2008.

Equation (5.6) in the microsimulation of costs described in the preceding chapters: Since we track the providers' cost over time, it is straightforward to compute the expenditures of those who adopt in the years during which the subsidy is available, then to compute how much the subsidy would cost from that information.

The benefit of the subsidy comes from increased savings, and it is computed as follows for the inpatient setting (with a similar calculation for the outpatient setting). In Chapter Three, we documented five forms of inpatient savings (see Table 3.1), each associated with the product of the three quantities $s_i$, $B_i$, and $N_i$ ($i=1, \ldots, 5$). The aggregate savings for the inpatient setting can therefore be described by the equation

$$S_t = \sum_{i=1}^{5} s_i B_i N_i = (p_t - p_{2004}) = \text{PS}^{\text{out}} \frac{p_t - p_{2004}}{1 - p_{2004}}, \tag{5.7}$$

where we have defined the total potential savings for the inpatient setting $\text{PS}^{\text{out}}$ (reported in Table 3.2) as

$$\text{PS}^{\text{out}} = \sum_{i=1}^{5} s_i B_i N_i (1 - p_{2004}). \tag{5.8}$$

The presence of the subsidy causes a stream of benefits over time, computed as the difference between the yearly savings with and without the subsidy. Using the superscript "sub" to denote the presence of the subsidy, the benefits of the subsidy are computed as follows:

$$B_t \equiv \text{PS}^{\text{out}} \frac{p_t^{\text{sub}} - p_t}{1 - p_{2004}}. \tag{5.9}$$

As a summary measure of benefits, we use the cumulative benefits over a time horizon $T$ (always 15 years in our case), which are defined as follows:

$$B \equiv \sum_{t=2004}^{2004+T-1} B_t. \tag{5.10}$$

Note that we add the sum over the entire period defined by the time horizon. Doing so underscores the fact that, even if a subsidy is limited in time, its effect lasts a long time (until $p_t^{\text{sub}} = p_t$), since it raises the level of adoption from the end of the subsidy on. Therefore, we defined benefit/cost ratios in terms of the cumulative benefit in Equation (5.10) and the total cost of the subsidy.

## Modeling Subsidies to Hospitals

We used the framework and the formulas above to model percentage subsidies to hospitals. We have used the total potential savings of $58.6 billion reported in Table (3.2) to quantify the value of the subsidy. We have performed a multi-way sensitivity analysis over a number of important parameters: the years in which the subsidy program begins (2006 or 2008), the price elasticity of demand (–0.25, –0.5, –0.75), the duration of the subsidy program (3 or 5 years), and the size of the subsidy (from 20 percent to 80 percent in 10-percent increments). We have reported the results of this analysis in the Excel spreadsheet inpatient_subsidy.xls.

As the above-mentioned parameters vary, a distribution of benefits and costs is obtained. In Figure 5.2, we report the cumulative distribution of the corresponding benefit/cost ratio. Obviously, the key parameter of this exercise is the elasticity $\varepsilon$, which has never been measured. For this reason, we have chosen a fairly large uncertainty interval for $\varepsilon$, between –0.75 and –0.25. The main point here is that, as shown in Figure 5.2, the benefit/cost ratio remains over 5 in more than 50 percent of the cases, and it is always above 1, even with the lowest value of elasticity.

It is important to understand under which conditions high benefit/cost ratios are achieved. A simple inspection of the spreadsheet inpatient_subsidy.xls shows that a key parameter is how soon the subsidy program starts. If the program is delayed, its cost-effectiveness drops quickly. For example, let us take the worst-case scenario of an elasticity equal to –0.25, and let us consider a 50-percent subsidy program that lasts for three years. If the subsidy starts in 2006, it costs about $7.5 billion, with a benefit/cost ratio of 4.2. However, if the program is delayed to year 2008, when adoption rates are higher, its costs balloon to $10.8 billion, with a benefit/cost ratio of only 2.4. This result is intuitive: The main reason that the benefit/cost ratios are high is that the benefits accumulate over time, and if we delay the start of the program, we cut the benefits while increasing the cost, since adoption rates are higher and demand for EMR-S is also higher.

Subsidies are also more cost-effective when they have short duration. Consider, again, an elasticity of –0.25 and a 50-percent subsidy starting in 2006: As we increase the duration from 3 to 5 years, the benefit/cost ratio drops from 4.2 to 3.

Finally, more-sizable subsidies tend to be more cost-effective. In fact, while cost increases more than linearly with size, benefit increases even faster. For example, consider an elasticity of –0.25 and a 3-year subsidy. As the size of the subsidy quadruples from 20 to 80 percent, the cost more than quadruples, going from $2.7 billion to $15.1 billion, but the benefit goes from $10 billion to $79.9 billion, with the benefit/cost ratio increasing from 3.7 to 5.3.

The general message, then, is that short-term subsidies that are reasonably sized tend to be preferable to smaller subsidies available for more years. For example,

**Figure 5.2**
**Distribution of the Benefit/Cost Ratio in the Multi-Way Sensitivity Analysis Reported in the Excel Spreadsheet inpatient_subsidy.xls**

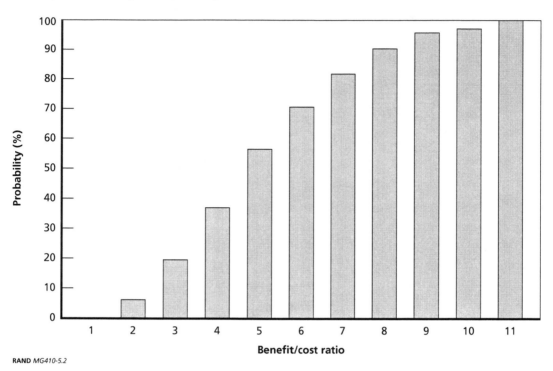

consider an elasticity of –0.25 and two subsidy programs that start in 2006: One program lasts three years, but covers 80 percent of the cost, and the other lasts five years and covers 40 percent of the cost. The total cost of these two programs is about the same, $15.1 billion for the first and $16.4 billion for the second, but the first program has a benefit/cost ratio of 5.3, whereas the second has a benefit/cost ratio of only 1.6.

In the spreadsheet inpatient_subsidy.xls, we report the total cost of a subsidy. It is instructive to put these figures in perspective by reporting how much it may cost to subsidize one hospital for a period of, say, four years. Using HCRIS hospital data (Centers for Medicare & Medicaid Services, 2005b), we considered all non-teaching hospitals with number of beds between 102 and 112 (this range is simply the median, 107, ±5). Using the cost model described in Chapter Four, we estimate that the average one-time cost of EMR-S for these hospitals is $3.8 million.[2] Assuming that the implementation of the EMR-S takes four years, consistent with Chapter Four, the 4-year cost of the EMR-S is the one-time cost plus some maintenance cost. Assuming that the maintenance cost is 30 percent of the portion of one-time cost al-

---

[2] The average operating expenses for these hospitals are about $25 million.

ready spent, the total cost of four years of EMR-S is $5.5 million. Using the occupancy figures for these hospitals, we computed that this amount would be covered in full by a subsidy of $81 per hospital bed day over four years.

## Modeling Per-Encounter Incentives for the Outpatient Setting

We have done some modeling of financial incentives for the outpatient setting. We assumed that a financial incentive program is established in year $T_{start}$ and lasts $n$ years. The financial incentive takes the following form: Physicians who adopt an EMR-S between year $T_{start}$ and year $T_{start}+n-1$ are given an amount $P$ per visit for $k$ years starting in the year they adopt (a reasonable choice would be $n=k=3$). Since we do not have the data to model the heterogeneity of physicians' behavior, we can only model an average physician, which allows us to translate the per-encounter incentive into a subsidy of the form of Equation (5.6).

Before we can proceed, we need to define cost $C$ appearing in Equation (5.6). The cost $C$ term certainly includes the one-time cost $C^{ot}$, as well as the discounted stream of future maintenance costs. We denote by $m_c$ the fraction of the one-time cost spent on maintenance each year (for example, $m_c$ was 20 percent in our calculations on cost of outpatient EMR-S). Then we can always write the present value of the discounted future stream of maintenance costs as $\gamma m_c C$, where $\gamma$ depends on the physician's discounting rate.

We do not have data on physicians' behavior that allow us to estimate the factor $\gamma$. From our reading of the literature, it seems that maintenance costs do not play a huge factor in the decision to acquire an EMR-S; therefore one could tentatively set $\gamma$ to 2, which is equivalent to saying that when the physician buys an EMR-S, he or she takes implicitly into account two years of maintenance.

If the maintenance cost does not seem too important, there is an additional cost to consider: Talking to some experts, it became clear that there is a hidden, "nonmonetary," cost in the acquisition of an EMR-S. This cost is not proportional to the one-time cost of the EMR-S; rather, it includes all the possible acquisition barriers. If we did not include this cost, then offering free EMR-S to all physicians would cause everybody to adopt an EMR-S immediately, which does not sound reasonable. We denote this cost by $C_0$, so that the cost $C$ of an EMR-S can be written as $C=C_0+C^{ot}(1+\gamma m_c)$.

The presence of the financial incentive brings to the physicians a revenue equal to $PVk$ (where $V$ is the average number of visits per year and $k$ is the number of years during which the physicians receive the payments[3]), which reduces the cost of

---

[3] We assume that $k$ is small, so we do not discount future income.

acquisition of the EMR-S. Using the same modeling approach that led us to Equation (5.6), we write the adoption curve under this incentive as

$$P_{t+1} = P_t + \frac{\alpha}{(C_0 + C^{ot}[1 + \gamma m_c] - PVk)^{|\varepsilon|}} \, p_t(1 - p_t). \tag{5.11}$$

The constant $\alpha$ is obtained by imposing the condition that, under no financial incentive ($P=0$), the adoption speed is equal to the parameter $b$ (in our simulations, $b=0.3$):

$$b = \frac{\alpha}{(C_0 + C^{ot}[1 + \gamma m_c])^{|\varepsilon|}}. \tag{5.12}$$

The final form of the adoption curve is then

$$P_{t+1} = P_t + b\left(1 - \frac{PVk}{C_0 + C^{ot}[1 + \gamma m_c]}\right)^{-|\varepsilon|} p_t(1 - p_t). \tag{5.13}$$

Note that by differentiating Equation (5.12) with respect to the price of an EMR-S, $C(1+\gamma m_c)$, we found that the price elasticity of demand for an EMR-S is not $\varepsilon$ but, rather,

$$\text{elasticity of demand} = \varepsilon \frac{C^{ot}(1 + \gamma m_c)}{C_0 + C^{ot}(1 + \gamma m_c)}. \tag{5.14}$$

The presence of the "nonmonetary" cost $C_0$ thus ensures that the price elasticity goes to 0 as the price of an EMR-S goes to 0. This characteristic of the model was introduced after a conversation with industry experts, who pointed out that even if the price of an EMR-S were reduced to 0, not all physicians would adopt one, and demand would stay bounded.

To provide the reader with the widest range of simulations of financial incentives of this type, we have implemented this model in the interactive Excel spreadsheet ambulatory_incentive_simulator.xls. The spreadsheet allows the user to vary interactively all the parameters used in this section, except for $\gamma$, which is set to 2.[4] The spreadsheet shows the adoption curves with and without the incentive, the cumulative benefits over 15 years, the total cost of the incentive, the cumulative

---

[4] The only relevant quantity is $C(1+\gamma m_c)$; therefore, a change in $\gamma$ can always be simulated by a change in $C$.

benefit/total-cost ratio, and the time evolution of the benefits of the incentives, as defined in Equation (5.9).

The spreadsheet is initialized by setting the one-time cost $C^{ot}$ at \$22,000, the maintenance cost at 20 percent of the one-time cost, the yearly number of visits $V$ equal to 3,000, the number of years during which the physician receives the incentive payment $k$ equal to 3 years, and the per-encounter payment $P$ equal to \$1.6. The per-encounter payment has been set to cover half of the cost of the EMR-S for a period of three years, assuming that the implementation time is two years. The calculation goes as follows:

**Year 1:** Since the implementation phase lasts two years, during the first year the physician spends half of the one-time cost—that is, \$11,000.
**Year 2:** In the second year, the physician spends the second half of the one-time cost (\$11,000), but also starts paying the maintenance cost on the already-existing equipment (valued at \$11,000). The maintenance cost is therefore $0.2 \times \$11,000 = \$2,200$. Total expenses in year 2 are therefore \$13,200.
**Year 3:** In the third year, the physician incurs the full maintenance cost, equal to \$4,400.

The total cost for the three years is \$28,600, which implies that the payment necessary to cover half of this amount is $\$28,600/(2kV) = \$28,600/(2 \times 3 \times 3,000) \approx \$1.6$. The cost of such an incentive payment is about \$2 billion. This amount also includes the assumption that half of the physicians who have adopted prior to year 2006 get a form of certification and become eligible for the incentive as well. The idea of a certification process has been introduced to make the scheme more realistic; it addresses a fairness issue that would arise if the incentive payment excluded early adopters.

The benefit/cost ratio associated with the parameters described above is 8.4, which is quite high. In general, we found that for a wide range of parameters, the benefit/cost ratio remains above 5. One of the most critical parameters is the year in which the subsidy begins: Since we are looking at a fixed horizon of 15 years, every year of delay causes a significant loss. The general lesson learned from experimenting with this simulator is that the most cost-effective incentives start very soon, last only a few years (say, 3) but are generous (say, 50 percent) while in place.

## Modeling a Price Change

Keeping everything else constant, an increase in demand for EMR-S, as projected by our adoption curves, would lead to an increase in the price of EMR-S. However, many factors control the price of EMR-S, and many industry experts seem to believe that prices of EMR-S will actually be going down in the near future. In addition, there might be government interventions, not necessarily in the form of subsidies to providers, aimed at lowering the price of EMR-S.

From a modeling point of view, a reduction in price is handled by Equation (5.6), the same that is used to model subsidies, where $X_t$ is interpreted as the percentage change in price for year $t$. Let us assume, for example, that we want to model a percentage reduction in price equal to $\delta$ (for example, $\delta=50$ percent), which takes place gradually over a period of $T_c$ years (starting in 2004, which is always our base year). In this case, the schedule $X_t$ would be

$$X_t = \begin{cases} \dfrac{\delta(t - 2004)}{T_c - 1} & 2004 \leq t \leq 2004 + T_c - 1 \\ \delta & t \geq 2004 + T_c - 1 \end{cases}.$$  (5.15)

We have modeled such a price change for the outpatient setting and have computed the benefits that would follow from the increased adoption, using Equations (5.9) and (5.10). An example of the size of the effect of the price change on the adoption curve is shown in Figure 5.3. Here, by *price* we mean the total cost of the EMR-S to the physician, which includes the one-time cost, the discounted stream of maintenance costs, and the "nonmonetary" cost.[5] Figure 5.3 refers to the case in which a price decrease of 50 percent takes place gradually over five years, starting in 2004. The price is assumed to remain constant at half the original level after the 5-year period. The elasticity of demand used for this simulation is –0.5.

Note that because adoption increases monotonically over time, the adoption curve with the price change continues to rise above the adoption curve without price change after the price has stabilized. On average over 15 years, adoption rates with the price change are 14.7 percent (or, equivalently, 8.8 percentage points) higher than those without the price change. The total benefit associated with the increased adoption is $29.6 billion.

To give an idea of how this number changes as a function of the size of the price change, the number of years it takes for the price change to take place, and the elasticity of demand, we have performed a simple three-way sensitivity analysis, which is reported in Table 5.1. As a rule of thumb, the benefits are almost linear in the elasticity, so reducing the elasticity from –0.5 to –0.25 halves the benefits. As noted before, it is in the nature of adoption phenomena that larger benefits are obtained by interventions that act sooner rather than later: For the same size of price change, a doubling of the time for the change to take place almost halves the benefits.

---

[5] Formally, *price* is defined as $C_t$ in Equation (5.4).

**Figure 5.3**
**Effect of a Reduction of 50 Percent in the Total Cost of Ambulatory EMR-S on Adoption Rates**

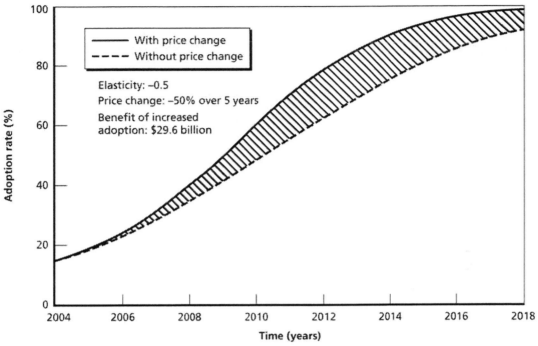

NOTE: The change takes place gradually over a period of five years, starting in the year 2004.
RAND *MG410-5.3*

**Table 5.1**
**Sensitivity Analysis for the National Benefit Associated with a Reduction in Total Cost of Ambulatory EMR-S**

| | Elasticity of demand: −0.5 | | | |
|---|---|---|---|---|
| Years for change to occur | Size of price change ($billions) | | | |
| | −15% | −25% | −35% | −50% |
| 5 | 7.3 | 12.8 | 19.2 | 29.6 |
| 7 | 6.2 | 11.1 | 16.2 | 24.5 |
| 10 | 4.5 | 8.5 | 12.1 | 18.6 |
| | Elasticity of demand: −0.25 | | | |
| Years for change to occur | Size of price change ($billions) | | | |
| | −15% | −25% | −35% | −50% |
| 5 | 3.9 | 7.1 | 9.8 | 15 |
| 7 | 3 | 5.6 | 7.7 | 13 |
| 10 | 2.1 | 4.3 | 6.3 | 9.4 |

# CHAPTER SIX

# Conclusion and Summary

In this document, we have presented several findings on the costs and benefits of HIT. We do not draw here the implications of these findings for policy; a discussion of HIT policy is presented in Taylor et al. (2005), nor do we attempt to set them against the larger background of how HIT is transforming healthcare, which is discussed in Hillestad et al. (2005). Rather, we summarize here the main lessons learned. We start with costs and benefits, whose main statistics are shown in Table 6.1.

Several messages emerge from this table:

- **Large benefits are associated with HIT adoption.** Summing over all sectors, we estimated about $40 billion in mean yearly savings, which correspond to potential savings of about $80 billion. Even with the wide uncertainty intervals shown in Figure 3.2, these are fairly large numbers, in absolute terms. However, we note that, on average, our percentage savings are quite small, between 10 and 15 percent. The savings, in absolute terms, are quite large, because the base cost—the level of national expenditures—is very high.
- **Benefits are substantially larger than costs.** It is sufficient to look at mean yearly savings. Summing over both the inpatient sector and the outpatient sec-

**Table 6.1**
**Summary of Benefits and Costs of EMR-S**

|  | Cost of EMR-S | | | HIT Savings | |
|---|---|---|---|---|---|
|  | Cumulative Cost ($billions) | One-Time Cost ($billions) | Mean Yearly Cost ($billions) (15 years) | Cumulative Savings ($billions) (15 years) | Mean Yearly Savings ($billions) (15 years) |
| Inpatient | 97.4 | 30.4 | 6.5 | 468.5 | 31.2 |
| Ambulatory | 17.2 | 7.3 | 1.1 | 159 | 10.6 |

tor, we obtained mean yearly benefits of about $40 billion, whereas we obtained mean yearly costs of $7.6 billion, for a benefit/cost ratio higher than 5. This ratio makes our findings very robust: Even if a large portion of the savings is not realized, the benefit/cost ratio would remain higher than 1. However, we note that our analysis is based on neither a best-case scenario nor a worst-case scenario: While there are reasons that lower savings might be realized, there also reasons that larger savings might be realized. We also note here that our analysis looked at only 10 sources of savings, and it does not include other sources of savings, such as reduction in emergency room expenditures or malpractice costs, nor at the potentially large savings brought by PACS in the inpatient setting.

- **Inpatient EMR-S are much more expensive than ambulatory EMR-S.** We found a great disparity between the inpatient and the outpatient settings in terms of costs: The mean yearly cost for the inpatient EMR-S is almost 6 times larger than the one for the outpatient setting. Ambulatory EMR-S turn out to be reasonably inexpensive when looked at on a national scale, with an annual cost per capita of about $3.7.

- **Most of the cumulative 15-year cost is due to maintenance costs.** We modeled maintenance costs as 30 percent and 20 percent of the one-time cost for inpatient and ambulatory EMR-S, respectively. This percentage implies that for the inpatient EMR-S, the maintenance cost is responsible for almost 70 percent of the cumulative cost, whereas for ambulatory EMR-S, this figure is 57 percent. It also implies that our cost estimates are quite sensitive to maintenance costs. Since we have been conservative with maintenance costs and have tried to err on the side of overestimation, it seems unlikely that our cost estimates are too low.

- **Savings to ambulatory EMR-S account for only one-fourth of the total savings, but they have better cost/benefit ratios than inpatient EMR-S.** Inasmuch as costs of inpatient EMR-S surpass costs of ambulatory EMR-S, savings in the outpatient setting are also much smaller than savings in the inpatient setting, accounting for only one-fourth of the total savings. However, ambulatory EMR-S are so much cheaper than inpatient EMR-S that the outpatient setting has the better cost/benefit ratio for mean yearly savings, equal to 9.1 (this ratio is 4.8 for the inpatient sector).

To provide a visual representation of some of these results, we show in Figure 6.1 how the net benefits (savings minus [−] costs) are expected to accrue over time. We see that in the first few years, the net benefits are very small, because of the delay between the beginning of the implementation and the full realization of savings. We report in these figures both the yearly and the cumulative net benefits: The latter are expected to reach, in 15 years, the value of $370 billion and $142 billion for the inpatient setting and outpatient setting, respectively. By that time, adoption is nearly

**Figure 6.1**
**Net Benefits (Savings – Costs) for Inpatient EMR-S and Outpatient EMR-S**

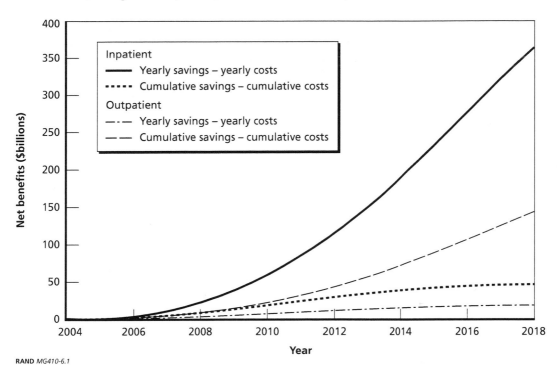

RAND *MG410-6.1*

complete, and the yearly savings are very close to the potential savings, while yearly costs are resulting almost exclusively from the maintenance costs.

Since we have documented quite large benefits from HIT adoption, it would seem reasonable to try to achieve those benefits sooner, incentivizing HIT adoption by artificially reducing the price of EMR-S. In our chapter on incentives, three main lessons were learned:

- It would be extremely valuable to design experiments aimed at estimating the instantaneous behavioral response of providers to a reduction in the EMR-S price. We relied on sensitivity analysis to show that, even under pessimistic conditions, incentives for HIT adoption have benefits that outweigh the costs. While this may be sufficient to make the case for considering incentive programs, even a rough estimate of the elasticity of demand for EMR-S would go a long way in helping to simulate more specific policy and budgetary scenarios.
- There are intrinsic reasons that incentives for adoption are likely to be cost-effective. Adoption of technology is a process with a long-term memory and a "contagious" nature. Not only is the effect of an exogenous shock remembered for a long time, since it puts the adoption curve forever above the previous levels, but it also can be greatly amplified: Each time a new provider adopts an

EMR-S, the probability that more providers will adopt the following year increases. These characteristics make HIT adoption a likely candidate for cost-effective incentives. In fact, a finite-duration incentive program may act on the adoption pattern for a short period but will have long-lasting effects, thanks to the amplification effect intrinsic in technology adoption. This explains why starting soon is a crucial condition for an incentive program to have a high benefit/cost ratio. Delaying the start of an incentive program to a time when adoption rates are already relatively high can be inefficiently expensive, because it may subsidize providers who would have adopted anyway. In addition, it leaves much less time for the benefits to accumulate over time, which is the main benefit of the incentive.

• Incentive programs are more likely to be cost-effective if they start early and do not last long, but are sizable. This is a corollary to the preceding statement. However, although the specific benefit/cost ratio of a program depends on the elasticity parameter $\varepsilon$ these conclusions are quite general and do not depend on it.

A fuller discussion of the findings on incentives is presented in Taylor et al. (2005), in which many of the numbers derived here are put in the context of making a case for a stronger involvement of the government in facilitating the spread of HIT adoption.

# Taxonomies

Each of the three taxonomies we constructed for classifying articles found in the literature and the individual findings extracted from those articles—on impacts, interventions, and HIT functionality—is defined in the following sections.

## Impacts

The Impacts taxonomy was derived from the Institute of Medicine–recommended aims for quality improvement in the healthcare system (Institute of Medicine, 2001). The first level included "Safe," "Effective," "Efficient," "Patient-Centered," "Timely," and "Equitable." Subordinate levels identified more-specific or topical items within the aims. For example, Safe included items such as "Reduce Adverse Drug Events" and "Reduce Complications." The full taxonomy is available in the spreadsheet HIT_Functional_Taxonomy.xls (worksheet "Impacts Taxonomy"). Findings were distributed among categories in the Impacts taxonomy as shown in Figure A.1.

In general, findings from the gray literature tended to focus on financial impacts of HIT, whereas those from peer-reviewed journals concerned safety and effectiveness, in addition to cost.

## Interventions

The Interventions taxonomy organized articles and findings according to the scope and type of organizational changes the projects were intended to bring about. Top-level headings in the taxonomy included

**Figure A.1**
**Distribution of Findings in the Impact Taxonomy**

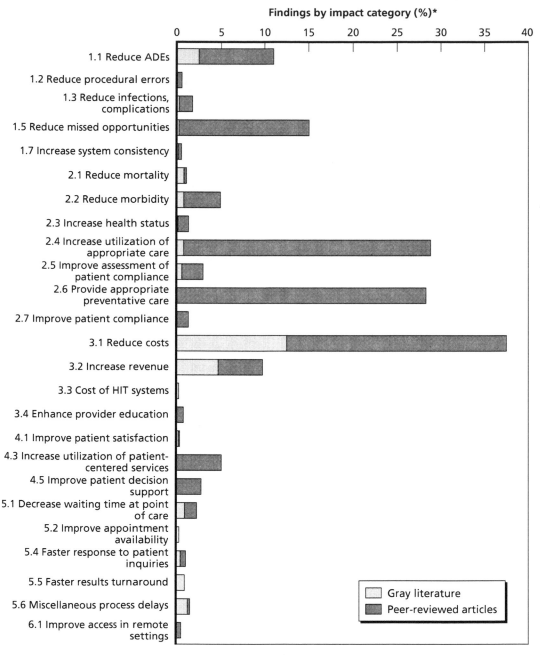

SOURCE: Authors' calculations based on literature search described in Chapter Two.
NOTES: Numbers are missing from those categories (e.g., 5.3) in which there were no findings.
*Total >100% reflects multiple impacts per finding.

1. Patient population management
2. Patient encounter/admission management
3. Administrative process management
4. Clinical process management
5. Community care management
6. Payer/insurer system management
7. National population health and health system management.

The complete taxonomy can be found in the spreadsheet HIT_Functional_Taxonomy.xls (worksheet "Interventions Taxonomy"). The distribution of findings for the peer-reviewed and gray literature is shown in Figure A.2.

Gray-literature findings tended to be clustered on issues of process management and patient-encounter management; peer-reviewed articles had a notable focus on population management, including prevention, error avoidance, and guidelines compliance.

## HIT Functionality Taxonomy

The Functionality taxonomy was the most detailed of the three taxonomies. It can be found on the spreadsheet HIT_Functional_Taxonomy.xls (worksheet "Features Taxonomy"). It was derived conceptually and substantively from early work of the HL7 Electronic Health Record Special Interest Group (Larsen et al., 2003). We added extra functions and system features by reviewing other sources, such as EMR products, consultant reports, the IOM letter report, among others. (A detailed list is available on the Utilities and References sheet of the taxonomy spreadsheet HIT_Functional_Taxonomy.xls).

The taxonomy was organized loosely on a process view of a typical patient encounter. It contains five levels: The first four are functional in that they refer to actions that the system performs or supports; the fifth level identifies features—i.e., characteristics of the systems that enable them to enact the functions. The top-level categories included the following:

**Figure A.2**
**Distribution of Findings in the Interventions Taxonomy for the Peer-Reviewed and Gray Literature**

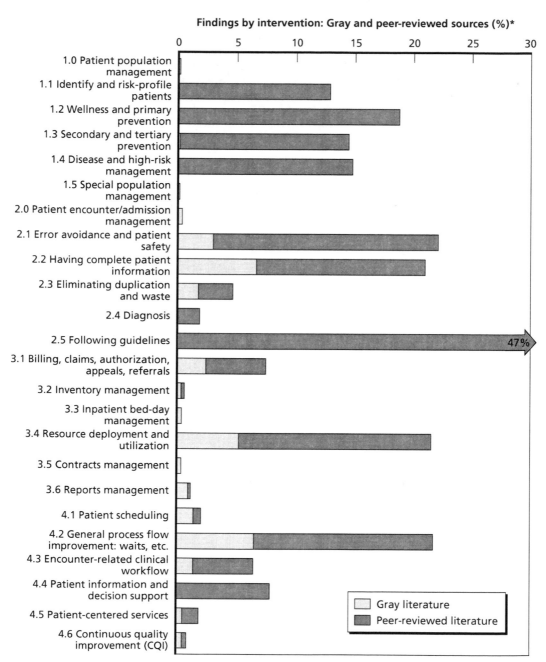

SOURCE: Authors' calculations based on literature search described in Chapter Two.
NOTE: Numbers refer to categories in the Intervention taxonomy.
*Total >100% reflects multiple impacts per finding.
RAND *MG410-A.2*

1.  Clinical operations
2.  Clinical assessment
3.  Clinical decisions
4.  Clinical orders
5.  Clinical actions, therapy
6.  Clinical documents
7.  Clinical communication and data management
8.  Clinical process change and improvement
9.  Administrative and financial functions
10. Implementing and managing information technology.

The distribution of findings at the second level of the Functional taxonomy is shown in Figure A.3. Findings clustered on viewing and entering data into patient records, and on order entry and care planning, with a host of ancillary functions mentioned.

**Figure A.3**
**Distribution of Findings at the Second Level of the Functional Taxonomy**

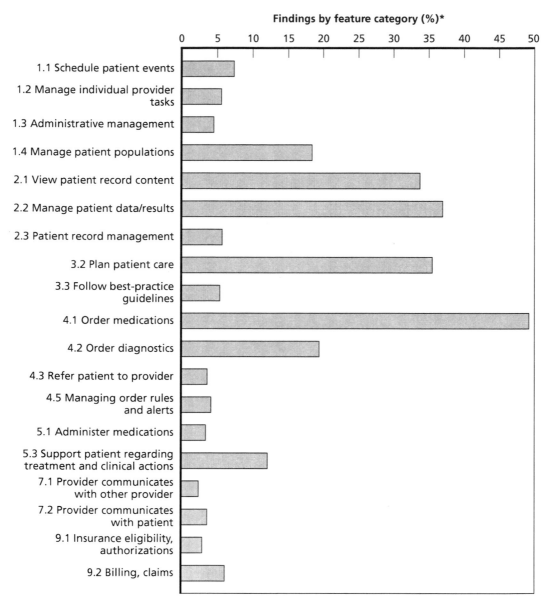

SOURCE: Authors' calculations based on literature search described in Chapter Two.
NOTE: Some item numbers (e.g., 3.1) may be missing because there were no findings in these categories.
*Total >100% reflects multiple features per finding.
RAND MG410-A.3

# A Note on Transaction and Administrative Costs

In Hillestad et al. (2005), we have focused on aspects of information technology pertaining to electronic medical records. However, it has long been recognized that information technology can play an important role in reducing healthcare administrative costs. Although a detailed examination of the potential savings in transaction costs from HIT is beyond the scope of this project, we attempted to identify a lower bound to this important source of savings.

A large body of work on this issue was performed more than a decade ago by the Workgroup for Electronic Data Interchange (WEDI, 1993). WEDI studied and quantified costs and benefits of standardized electronic data interchange (EDI) in healthcare. We summarize some of their findings on the potential savings in transaction costs in Table B.1. All the figures are in billions of 2004 dollars, converted using the Consumer Price Index.

**Table B.1**
**Summary of Savings in Transaction Costs Estimated by WEDI (1993)**

| Transaction | Lower Bound | Higher Bound | Mean |
|---|---|---|---|
| Claims Submission | 5.9 | 17.2 | 11.5 |
| Enrollment | 2.8 | 5.7 | 4.2 |
| Payment and Remittance | 1.4 | 1.7 | 1.6 |
| Eligibility | 0.3 | 0.6 | 0.5 |
| Claims Inquiry | 0.4 | 0.5 | 0.4 |
| Materials Management | 3.9 | 5.9 | 4.9 |
| Prescription Ordering | 0.9 | 0.9 | 0.9 |
| Coordination of Benefits | 0.6 | 0.9 | 0.7 |
| Test Order/Result | 0.4 | 0.4 | 0.4 |
| Referral/Authorization | 0.2 | 0.2 | 0.2 |
| Appointing/Scheduling | 0.1 | 0.1 | 0.1 |
| Total | 16.9 | 34.0 | 25.5 |

NOTE: Values are in billions of 2004 dollars.

The savings figures in the table are obviously dated and cannot be used. They should be adjusted downward because adoption rates have increased since 1993, at least for some important items, such as claims submission and processing; therefore, we should not count those who have adopted in this period. However, both volume of transactions and prices have been increasing in the past decade; therefore, we should adjust the savings upward. It is not obvious which of these two effects may dominate.

By analyzing and updating the two large sources of potential transaction savings identified by WEDI in 1993 (claims submission and enrollment), we identified $12.5 billion in potential annual savings. Of these savings, $11 billion come from electronic claims processing and $1.5 billion from online enrollment. Although electronic claims processing can occur without providers having adopted an Electronic Medical Record System (EMR-S), it requires providers or their contracted billing intermediary to convert clinical and administrative patient care information into the proper electronic format for submission to payers. The use of EMR-S greatly facilitates this process by making electronic clinical care and administrative data available to the system's practice management and billing software to generate and transmit electronic claims. For those providers without this technology that currently submit electronic claims from a freestanding practice management system or through an intermediary, this process could eliminate the paper-based and office staff components of that process, as well as intermediaries' charges, creating savings not included in our lower-bound estimate.

For those providers adopting EMR-S and newly initiating electronic billing directly, this represents a new transaction efficiency savings that we have attempted to estimate, as well as improved cash flow to providers (the value of which is not included in our savings estimate). In addition, the trade press reports that electronic claims from EMR-S are more likely to be complete and accurate, reducing the rate of requests for further justification, denials, and appeals (the costs of which we did not include in our lower bound estimate of transaction savings). Finally, our discussion with executives at Trizetto, a leading e-health company, and our reading of the industry press suggest a wide range of other potential HIT-enabled transaction savings, including electronic confirmation of coverage, medical-necessity authorization, real-time cost-sharing calculations at the point of care, automatic payments from health savings accounts, real-time identification of preferred providers or therapies/drugs, real-time authorization of referrals, and a range of online administrative support services that eliminate the necessity for patient or provider phone calls and delays. Each of these, and a number of other sources identified by WEDI, could decrease the volume of unnecessary transactions and increase transaction efficiency, resulting in additional savings not included in our lower-bound estimate.

Additional research is needed in this area to update the 1993 WEDI study. However, for the purpose of this monograph, we are quite confident in saying that the lower bound of potential savings in transaction costs from providers implementing EMR-S and electronically interfacing with payers is greater than $10 billion per year. The details of our calculations are presented in the next section.

## Claims Submission

### How Many Claims?

The most recent estimate we found for the total number of claims filed every year in the United States is 6 billion (*Health Data Directory*, 2000). The number of Medicare claims is well known and was set at 1 billion in 2004.[1] To check that our estimates are consistent, we note that Medicare accounts for 17.5 percent of national health expenditures: A trivial extrapolation suggests, then, that the number of claims should be about 5.7 billion, which is reasonably close to the 6-billion figure given above.

### How Many Claims Are Processed Electronically?

Gillette (2003) gives two estimates for the percentage of electronically processed claims, 60 and 70 percent, obtained from different sources, whereas the WEDI report sets it at 15 percent in the year 1992 (WEDI, 1993). Ober (2000) sets this number in 2000 at 68 percent, up from 61 percent in 1998. According to Goedert (1996), this number was 41.5 percent in 1994 and 47 percent in 1995. Danzon and Furukawa (2001) reported that the Faulkner & Gray *1999 Health Data Directory* sets this figure at 62 percent. These data are reported in Figure B.1.

Given the data above, we take the current percentage of claims processed electronically to be 70 percent. However, virtually all Medicare claims are processed electronically now (http://www.cms.hhs.gov/charts/series/sec2.pdf), which implies that the percentage of non-Medicare claims processed electronically is 64 percent, leaving 1.8 billion claims processed manually. Here, we focus on non-Medicare claims, because Medicare claims have almost full adoption and, so, we cannot expect much additional savings; also, Medicare has very small administrative costs.

---

[1]  See www.cms.hhs.gov/medicarereform/contractingreform/odf/mma911_odf_slides.pdf.

**Figure B.1**
**Time Evolution of the Percentage of Claims That Are Processed Electronically**

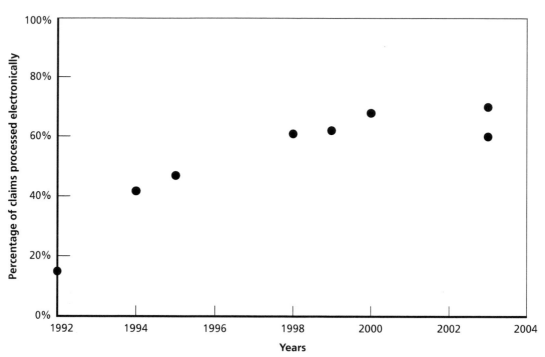

SOURCES: Gillette (2003), WEDI (1993), Ober (2000), Goedert (1996), and Danzon and Furukawa (2001).
RAND MG410-B.1

## Cost and Savings per Claim

A number of sources give different values for paper-claims filing:

- DeJesus (2000) sets the cost of filing a paper claim at $11. In the same paper, an industry expert is quoted as reporting savings of 90 percent obtained by switching to electronic claims.
- According to Quinn (2003), the cost of filing a paper claim was $7 to $12 in 2003; if the filing were done electronically, $5.5 to $9 would be saved per claim, which implies savings of about 75 percent.
- Gillette (2003) reports several figures. The cost of filing a paper claim is set between $4 and $8, with two sources reporting savings of 20 percent and 50 percent, respectively.
- Phelan (2003) reports a table that details different steps in claim processing and the savings that can be achieved at each step. The total cost of the claim is set at $7, with savings of $4.7 (67-percent savings).

- Danzon and Furukawa (2001) and Rouse and Chalson (2000) reported that the cost per claim is between $10 and $15, whereas the cost of an electronic claim is between $2 and $4, implying savings of about 76 percent.

Averaging all these results, we found a saving of 63 percent over an average cost of each claim of $9.8 (all values have been converted to 2004 dollars). Using the 5-billion figure for non-Medicare claims, with a 64-percent adoption rate for electronic claims, we obtained a figure of 1.8 billion claims filed on paper, which corresponds to an expenditure of $17.6 billion, out of which we could save 63 percent. Therefore, we conclude that the potential savings from electronic-claims processing is about $11 billion.

## Enrollment

Health plans could save substantial amounts by switching from manual, paper-based enrollment to electronic, Web-based procedures. We do not have hard data on how much it costs for a health plan to enroll one individual. We do have an estimate from Trizetto, which sets the cost of paper-based enrollment at $18 to $25 per member per year (http://www.trizetto.com/release/eenroll.asp). Trizetto suggests that enrollment could be cut (at least) in half, saving $9 to $12.5 per member per year. A recent estimate of the number of people covered by employer-sponsored plans, from the Kaiser Family Foundation website, is 54 percent (for 2003). Applying this percentage to the most recent Bureau of Census population estimate, we obtain 159 million people, which translates into a savings of $1.4 billion to $2 billion per year, for an average of $1.5 billion. Since we have yet to find evidence of widespread adoption of online enrollment, we take the percentage of current adopters to be negligible, which implies that the potential savings are $1.5 billion.

To see whether this estimate is credible, we make the assumption of savings from reduced labor, which translates this figure into FTEs saved. From the National Compensation Survey of the Bureau of Labor Statistics, the total hourly compensation, in 2004, for service occupations in the healthcare and social assistance sector is $14.46 (virtually the same for insurance claims and policy processing clerks). Under the usual assumption of 52 working weeks, we find that $1.5 billion corresponds to 49,872 FTEs. This number is reasonable when compared with the number of FTEs saved reported by the WEDI group, which is between 85,000 and 171,000.

## Conclusions

Looking at only two sources of savings, electronic-claims processing and online enrollment, we found $12.5 billion in potential savings, which justifies the statement that savings in transaction costs should exceed $10 billion.

# Cost of Connectivity

*Connectivity* is the infrastructure necessary to allow entities belonging to the healthcare system to share patients' clinical information. The only well-documented example of such a system is the Santa Barbara County Data Exchange (Brailer et al., 2003), although cost data for this project are not available. What is available is the financial analysis developed by McKinsey & Company, which consists of a set of models and scenarios (Brailer et al., 2003). In the following sections, we use that analysis as a baseline for estimating how much it would cost to "connect" the entire country. Once a national estimate has been obtained, we use alternative data to validate it, or at least to validate parts of the computation. These estimates are subject to much uncertainty, starting from the fact that no clear definitions of connectivity exist. One expert in the field suggested that these might be lower bounds and that the true cost could be twice as high.

First, we describe the cost reported in the Santa Barbara example (Brailer et al., 2003), then we use two alternative methods for scaling up the Santa Barbara model to national-level estimates.

## Costs from the Santa Barbara County Demonstration

The financial analysis of costs and benefits describes different scenarios and computes costs and benefits for each scenario. The scenarios correspond to regions of different sizes (small, medium, and large) and to two different levels of penetration of connectivity (low and high).[1] The definitions of the scenarios are reported in Table C.1, and the costs include:

- integration of systems
- deployment of central data-sharing services

---

[1] By *penetration,* we mean the extent to which different entities are connected to each other.

- development and validation of algorithms for generation and maintenance of a master patient list
- training physicians and their offices
- supporting the implementation and operation of the central oversight entities.

The costs corresponding to the different scenarios are reported in Table C.2.

In addition to the cost per region, the study also reports the *cost per constituent*, which is shown in Table C.3. These figures refer to a large region with high penetration; figures for the other scenarios are not provided. This limitation will force us to assume, later in this appendix, that the cost per constituent does not vary with the size of the region. Note that the Pharmacy Benefits Manager (PBMs) are missing from the list of constituents.

**Table C.1**
**The Scenarios Considered in the Santa Barbara County Financial Analysis**

| Region Size | Constituent Type | Total Number in Region | Penetration | |
|---|---|---|---|---|
| | | | Low | High |
| Large | | | | |
| | Major hospital | 10 | 3 | 7 |
| | Diagnostic imaging center | 5 | 2 | 4 |
| | Independent laboratory | 3 | 1 | 2 |
| | PBMs | 5 | 1 | 3 |
| | Major physicians groups | 5 | 1 | 3 |
| | Physicians | 5,000 | 750 | 1,750 |
| Medium | | | | |
| | Major hospital | 6 | 2 | 4 |
| | Diagnostic imaging center | 2 | 1 | 2 |
| | Independent laboratory | 1 | 1 | 1 |
| | PBMs | 5 | 1 | 3 |
| | Major physicians groups | 2 | 1 | 2 |
| | Physicians | 1,000 | 150 | 350 |
| Small | | | | |
| | Major hospital | 1 | 1 | 1 |
| | Diagnostic imaging center | 1 | 1 | 1 |
| | Independent laboratory | 1 | 0 | 1 |
| | PBMs | 5 | 0 | 3 |
| | Major physicians groups | 0 | 1 | 0 |
| | Physicans | 200 | 30 | 70 |

SOURCE: Brailer et al. (2003).
NOTES: *Penetration* is the extent to which different entities are connected to each other.
PBM = Pharmacy Benefits Manager.

**Table C.2**
**The Costs Corresponding to the Different
Scenarios in the Santa Barbara County
Demonstration**

| Region Size | Connectivity Penetration | |
| --- | --- | --- |
| | Low | High |
| Large | $1,000,000 | $2,200,000 |
| Medium | 800,000 | 1,400,000 |
| Small | 490,000 | 780,000 |

SOURCE: Brailer et al. (2003).

**Table C.3**
**The Cost of Connectivity per Healthcare
Constituent: Large Region, High Penetration**

| Constituent | Cost |
| --- | --- |
| Hospital | $120,000 |
| Imaging Center | $110,000 |
| Laboratory | $110,000 |
| Physician Group | $120,000 |
| Solo Physician | $40 |

Now, we analyze these data in two different ways.

## Scaling Up: Method 1

An obvious way to produce national-level estimates of the cost of connectivity is to take the cost per constituent and multiply it by the total number of constituents in the United States. However, we also need to exclude from the calculations the number of constituents that are already connected in systems such as the Santa Barbara County Data Exchange. Current evidence suggests that this number is very small, and we disregard this effect. In the following paragraphs, we present national numbers for each constituent.

### Hospitals
According to the AHA website, in 2003 there were 5,764 registered hospitals.

## Imaging Centers

We searched several sources for the current number of imaging centers in the United States. The data we found are plotted in Figure C.1. The SMG Marketing Group and Verispan compile a directory of diagnostic imaging centers, whose latest edition has 5,475 entries (Verispan/SMG Marketing Group, 2004). This number seems to be well in accord with the observed growth trend of the past few years (SMG Marketing Group, 2000; Aunt Minnie, 2002; AGFA, 2004; Norbut, 2004; Chandler, 2004; Wiley, 2004; Verispan/SMG Marketing Group, 2004).

## Laboratories

The most quoted source of data about the laboratory testing industry we found is Marketdata Enterprises (2002a). According to this source, there are 4,500 to 5,000 independent commercial laboratories, 6,100 hospital labs, and 99,000 physician's office labs. We need to count only the independent labs for our purposes. The figure on independent labs agrees with the 5,000 figure given by Kenneth Freeman of Quest Diagnostics in an interview (Pontius, 2002).

**Figure C.1**
**Number of Imaging Centers in the United States**

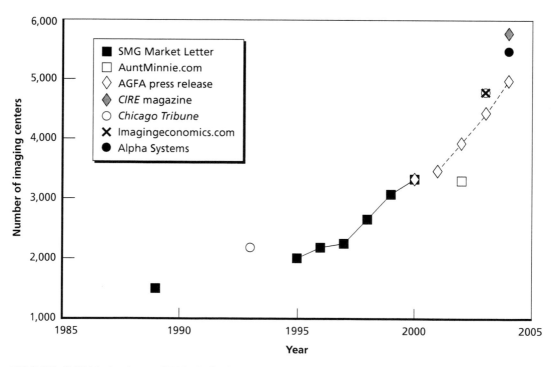

SOURCES: SMG Market Letter (SMG Marketing Group, 2000), AuntMinnie.com (Aunt Minnie, 2002), AGFA (2004), *CIRE (Commercial Investments Real Estate)* magazine (Norbut, 2004), *Chicago Tribune* (Chandler, 2004), Imaging Economics (Wiley, 2004), Alpha Systems (Verispan/SMG Marketing Group, 2004).

**Physicians**

Unfortunately, the Santa Barbara study (Brailer et al., 2003) does not define "physician group"; therefore, we do not know the multiplier needed to scale up this cost to the national level. However, the report performs an analysis for "regions" of different sizes, defined by a given number of constituents (a large region has seven hospitals, four imaging centers, two laboratories, three physician groups, and 1,750 solo physicians). The cost numbers are given for a region of large size. For such a region, the total cost of connectivity to physicians is 51 percent of the cost to hospitals. Therefore, the national-level estimate of the cost of connectivity to physicians will be set equal to 51 percent of the cost to hospitals.

As noted above, Table C.3 does not include the cost of PBMs, and PBMs have not been included in any of the other categories. If we take the definition of a large region and sum up the cost for the constituents, we obtain $1,930,000, instead of $2,200,000. We attribute this difference of $270,000 to the missing PBMs. To scale up this number, we used the same strategy we used for physicians and note that the PBM cost is 32 percent of the cost to hospitals. At the national level, we estimated that cost to hospitals as $704 million; therefore, we estimated that the PBM cost at the national level is $225 million.

We conclude that the total cost of connectivity at the national level is about $2.4 billion, divided among constituents as shown in Table C.4.


## Scaling Up: Method 2

An alternative method for producing a national-level estimate relies exclusively on Tables C.1 and C.2. If we know how many "small," "medium," and "large" regions are in the United States, we can multiply these numbers by the corresponding costs and have an estimate of the cost of connectivity for the entire country.

To use this strategy, we make the following assumptions:

1. "Regions" correspond to U.S. counties.
2. The size of a region (county) is determined by the number of hospitals in that region, even if it is defined also in terms of the number of imaging centers, laboratories, PBMs, and physicians.

We used the 2000 *Area Resource File* (ARF), available at www.arfsys.com, to obtain the number of hospitals for each U.S. county. The distribution of the number

**Table C.4**
**The Estimated Cost of Connecting All U.S. Facilities in an Approach Similar to That for Santa Barbara County**

| Constituent | Cost per Constituent ($) | Number of Constituents | National Cost ($millions) |
|---|---|---|---|
| Hospital | 120,000 | 5,864 | 704 |
| Imaging center | 110,000 | 5,475 | 602 |
| Laboratory | 110,000 | 5,000 | 550 |
| Physicians | | | 359 |
| PBMs | | | 225 |
| Total | | | 2,440 |

SOURCE: Authors' calculations based on Brailer et al. (2003).

**Figure C.2**
**Distribution of the Number of Hospitals per County**

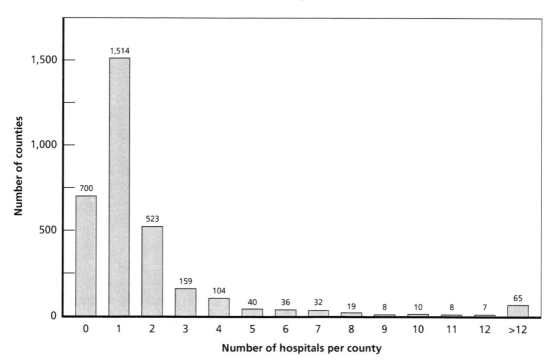

SOURCE: *Area Resource File* (ARF), www.arfsys.com.

RAND *MG410-C.2*

of hospitals per county is shown in Figure C.2, where we report on the vertical axis the number of counties with 1, 2, . . . , $n$ hospitals. Note that there are 700 counties with no hospitals: We can assume that these counties will not be connected at all, leading to lower cost estimates, or that they will be connected as every other "small" county, leading to higher estimates.

In Table C.1, small regions have one hospital, medium regions have six hospitals, and large regions have 10 hospitals. We needed to extend the definitions so that we could assign a size to each county. We computed the results for different choices of cutoff values as follows (where the numbers in parenthesis denote alternative cutoff values used for the sensitivity analysis):

- **Small county:** if the number of hospitals is less than or equal to 2 (3)
- **Medium county:** if the number of hospitals is greater than or equal to 3 (4) and less than or equal to 8 (9)
- **Large county:** if the number of hospitals is greater than or equal to 9 (10).

Now that we can assign a size to each county, we simply count the number of counties in each size category, assign them the corresponding cost from Table C.2, and sum the costs over all the counties. The result is fairly insensitive to the choice of the cutoffs that define the size. Different cutoff choices lead to results in the $2.25-billlion to $2.37-billion range. If we include the counties with no hospitals and assign them in the category "small," we need to add an extra $0.55 billion. *Therefore, our final estimate for the cost of connectivity is in the range $2.25 billion–2.92 billion, with an average of $2.6 billion.* Note that this estimate is very close to the one obtained using method 1.

## Validation

- From a conversation with a former CEO of an institution dedicated to information exchange, we know that the 14 hospitals associated with that institution spent $2 million–$2.5 million on information and data exchange, which is equivalent to $143,000–$179,000 per hospital. If we scale up this figure, we obtain a cost of connectivity to hospitals in the $824-million–$1,032-million range.
- A report of the Patient Safety Institute (PSI) (Emerging Practices First Consulting Group, 2004) mentions that the cost to build a national PSI infrastructure is approximately $2.5 billion. According to PSI, "The PSI network enables real time access to clinical information at the point of care or decision."

- Winona Health Online is another example of a connected community. Uehling (2001), a Cerner representative, quotes the following costs for a city that wants to imitate Winona:

  - Setup of website: $ 50,000 to $150,000
  - Connecting physicians to system: $5,000 to $25,000 per location
  - Consumer fee: $25 per user for the first year; $15 thereafter.

Uehling further suggests that the first year may cost $150,000–$400,000. Maintenance fees range from $50,000 to $150,000 annually. These numbers are on the high side, compared to the cost per constituent seen in Santa Barbara. Given that Winona is a community of 27,000 people, the cost per person for the first year is in the $5.5–$14.8 range ($10 per person, on average). If we apply the $10-per-person figure to the county of Santa Barbara, we obtain about $4 million. This figure is large compared with the estimated $2.2 million of a "large" region. However, it is not too large if we apply it to the entire U.S. population, because we obtain $2.9 billion.

## Conclusion

Using the results of our two calculations, we conclude that the cost of implementing a Santa Barbara–like system across the United States is about $2.5 billion. This cost should be spread over time as HIT is adopted, and maintenance costs should be added to it. If we assume that our current level of connectivity is low (5 percent) and that maintenance costs are 30 percent of the fixed cost, we can use Equation (2.3) to find that, over the next 15 years, the cumulative cost of connectivity will be $6 billion, for a mean yearly cost of $0.4 billion. As stated in the introduction to this appendix, one expert of the sector suggested that this might be a lower bound and that the true cost might be twice as high.

# Bibliography

AGFA, "AGFA Introduces Comprehensive RIS Solution for Rapidly Growing Imaging Center Market in U.S. and Canada," Mortsel, Belgium, 2004. Available online at http://www.agfa.com/canada/en/news/news_tcm98-5950.jsp (as of February 14, 2005).

American Hospital Association, *The State of Hospitals' Financial Health,* Chicago, Ill., 2002. Available online at http://www.aha.org/aha/advocacy-grassroots/advocacy/advocacy/content/Wp2002HospFinances.doc (as of February 14, 2005).

American Medical Association, ed., *Physician Characteristics and Distribution in the US, 2005,* Chicago, Ill., 2005.

Anderson, M. R., "Extensive Evaluation Ranks Top Electronic Medical Record Applications," Montgomery, Texas: AC Group, Inc., 2004. Available online at http://www.acgroup.org (as of February 14, 2005).

*Area Resource File (ARF),* http://www.arfsys.com.

Atlantic Imaging Group, Cedar Knolls, N.J.: technical report, 2005. Available online at http://www.aignetwork.com/Downloads/Brochure.pdf (as of February 14, 2005).

Audet, A., et al., "Information Technologies: When Will They Make It into Physicians' Black Bags?" *Medscape General Medicine,* Vol. 6, No. 4, 2004.

Aunt Minnie, "AuntMinnie.com Launches New Resource Focused on Diagnostic Imaging Centers," Tucson, Arizona, 2002. Available online at http://www.auntminnie.com/index.asp?Sec=abt\&Sub=prs\&Pag=dis\&ItemId=55782 (as of February 14, 2005).

Baldwin, F., "CPRs in the Winner's Circle: Award-Winning Organizations Set New Standards of Care with Electronic Data Capture," *Healthcare Informatics,* 2003.

Bates, D., and D. Boyle, "What Proportion of Common Diagnostic Tests Appear Redundant?" *JAMA,* Vol. 104, No. 4, 1998, pp. 361–368.

Bigelow, J., et al., "Technical Executive Summary in Support of 'Can Electronic Medical Record Systems Transform Healthcare?' and 'Promoting Health Information Technology'," *Health Affairs,* Web Exclusive, September 14, 2005a.

Bigelow, J., K. Fonkych, C. Fung, and J. Wang, *Analysis of Healthcare Interventions That Change Patient Trajectories,* Santa Monica, Calif.: RAND Corporation, MG-408-HLTH, 2005b.

Bingham, A., "A Computerized Patient Records Benefit Physician Offices," *Healthcare Financial Management,* 1997.

Bower, A., *The Diffusion and Value of Healthcare Information Technology,* Santa Monica, Calif.: RAND Corporation, MG-272-HLTH, 2005.

Brailer, D., N. Augustinos, L. Evans, et al., *Moving Toward Electronic Health Information Exchange: Interim Report on the Santa Barbara County Data Exchange,* Oakland, Calif.: California HealthCare Foundation, 2003.

Buerhaus, P. I., D. Staiger, and D. Auerbach, "Implications of an Aging Registered Nurse Workforce," *JAMA,* Vol. 283, No. 22, 2000, pp. 2948–2954.

Buerhaus, P. I., D. Staiger, and D. Auerbach, "Is the Current Shortage of Hospital Nurses Ending?" *Health Affairs,* Vol. 22, No. 6, 2003, pp. 191–198.

Bureau of Health Professions (BHP), *Projected Supply, Demand and Shortages of Registered Nurses: 2000–2020,* Washington, D.C.: Health Resources and Services Administration, 2002. Available online at ftp://ftp.hrsa.gov/bhpr/nationalcenter/rnproject.pdf (as of February 14, 2005).

Cap Gemini Ernst & Young, *Financial Impact Analysis on Pharmacy Risk Pools,* 2000. Available online at http://www.allscripts.com/ahcs/epres/epres.pdf (as of February 14, 2005).

Cap Gemini Ernst & Young, *Research by Cap Gemini Ernst & Young US LLC: E-Prescribing in a Multi-Center Group,* 2004. Available online at http://www.allscripts.com/ahcs/news_2.asp?S=2017\&ID=2 (as of February 14, 2005).

Carey, K., "Hospital Length of Stay and Cost: A Multilevel Modeling Analysis," *Health Services & Outcomes Research Methodology,* Vol. 3, 2002, pp. 41–56.

CCA Medical, *Rocky Mount Family Medical Center Slashes Transcription Costs Using ChartWare,* Greenville, S.C., 2005. Available online at http://www.ccamedical.com/rmfmc.html (as of May 22, 2005).

Centers for Medicare & Medicaid Services, *National Health Expenditures,* Baltimore, Md., 2005a. Available online at http://www.cms.hhs.gov/statistics/nhe/ (as of February 14, 2005).

Centers for Medicare & Medicaid Services, *Healthcare Cost Report Information System (HCRIS) Dataset,* Baltimore, Md., 2005b. Available online at http://www.cms.hhs.gov/data/download/hcris_hha/readme_09_30_04.asp (as of February 14, 2005).

Centers for Medicare & Medicaid Services, *Market Basket Data and Related Products,* Baltimore, Md., 2005c. Available online at http://www.cms.hhs.gov/statistics/market-basket/pps-hospital.asp (as of February 14, 2005).

Chandler, S., "Body-Scan Industry Weakens: Economy, Lack of Doctor Support May Prove Fatal," *Chicago Tribune,* 2004.

Cooper Pediatrics, *Primary Care Davies Award,* 2003. Available online at http://www.himss.org/content/files/davies_2003_primarycare_cooper.pdf (as of May 22, 2005).

Danzon, P., and M. Furukawa, "Health Care: Competition and Productivity," *The Economic Payoff from the Internet Revolution,* Washington, D.C.: Brookings Institution Press, 2001, Chapter 7.

DeJesus, E., "Claims Processing Speeds Up," *Healthcare Informatics,* 2000.

Ellingsen, G., and E. Monteiro, "Big Is Beautiful. Electronic Patient Records in Norway 1980–2000," *Methods of Information in Medicine,* Vol. 42, 2003. Available online at http://www.idi.ntnu.no/~ericm/methods.subm.pdf (as of May 31, 2005).

Emerging Practices First Consulting Group, *Economic Value of a Community Clinical Information Sharing Network,* Plano, Texas: Patient Safety Institute, 2004.

Fickel, K., "Hot-Wiring Hospitals," *Profit Magazine,* 2001. Available online at http://www.oracle.com/oramag/profit/01-nov/p41industry.html (as of May 31, 2005).

Fonkych, K., and R. Taylor, *The State and Pattern of Health Information Technology Adoption,* Santa Monica, Calif.: RAND Corporation, MG-409-HLTH, 2005.

Gillette, B., "Federal Regs Spur Total Electronic Claims Processing," *Managed Healthcare Executive,* Vol. 13, No. 4, 2003.

Goedert, J., "1995—A Healthy Year for Electronic Claims Growth," *Health Data Management,* Vol. 4, No. 1, 1996.

*Health Data Directory,* Faulkner & Gray, 2000.

Healthcare Information and Management Systems Society (HIMSS), *HIMSS Analytics Database* (formerly the *Dorenfest IHDS+ Database*), Chicago, Ill.: 2004.

Health Strategies Group, *Hospital Pharmacy Trends Summary,* Lambertville, N.J., second release, 2004. Available online at http://www.healthstrats.com/download/document.cfm?d=1535 (as of February 14, 2005).

Heffler, S., et al., "Health Spending Projections Through 2013," *Health Affairs,* 2004, pp. W4-79–W4-93. Available online at http://content.healthaffairs.org/cgi/reprint/hlthaff.w4.79v1 (as of February 14, 2005).

Hillestad, R., J. Bigelow, A. Bower, et al., "Can Electronic Medical Record Systems Transform Healthcare? Potential Health Benefits, Savings, and Costs," *Health Affairs,* Vol. 24, No. 5, September 14, 2005.

HSM Group Ltd., "Acute Care Hospital Survey of RN Vacancy and Turnover Rates in 2000," *Journal of Nursing Administration,* Vol. 32, No. 9, 2002, pp. 437–439.

Institute of Medicine (IOM), ed., *Crossing the Quality Chasm: A New Health System for the 21st Century,* Washington, D.C.: National Academy Press, 2001.

Johnston, D., et al., *The Value of Computerized Provider Order Entry in Ambulatory Setting,* Boston, Mass.: Center for Information Technology Leadership, Partners HealthCare, 2003.

Kane, C., *The Practice Arrangements of Patient Care Physicians, 2001,* Chicago, Ill.: American Medical Association, Center for Policy Research, 2004. Available online at http://www.ama-assn.org/ama1/pub/upload/mm/363/pmr-022004.pdf (as of February 14, 2005).

Kane, N., and R. Siegrist, *Understanding Rising Hospital Inpatient Costs: Key Components of Cost and The Impact of Poor Quality,* Chicago, Ill.: Blue Cross Blue Shield, 2002. Available online at www.bcbs.com/coststudies/reports/4_Inpatient_Qual_Assess.pdf (as of February 14, 2005).

Larsen, E., G. Dickinson, L. Fischetti, et al., *The EHR Systems Functional Model and Standard Initiative,* Ann Arbor, Mich.: Health Level Seven, 2003. Available online at www.hl7.org/ehr/documents/public/documents/HL7_EHR_Functional_Model.doc (as of February 14, 2005).

MacDonald, K., and J. Metzger, *Achieving Tangible IT Benefits in Small Physician Practices,* Oakland, Calif.: California Health Care Foundation, 2002.

Marketdata Enterprises, *The U.S. Medical Laboratories Industry,* Tampa, Fla.: 2002a.

Marketdata Enterprises, "Strong Growth Resumes for Clinical Lab Testing Industry, as Role Expands Beyond Diagnosis Only," Press Release, Tampa, Fla., 2002b. Available online at http://www.mkt-data-ent.com/pressreleases/Medical_Labs_Industry_PR_03-07-2003.doc (as of February 14, 2005).

MedicaLogic, *Ambulatory EMR: Establishing a Business Case, White Paper,* 2004. Available online at http://www.medicalogic.com/download/www/emr/whitepapers/business_case.pdf (as of May 22, 2005).

Mekhjian, H., et al., "Immediate Benefits Realized Following Implementation of Physician Order Entry at an Academic Medical Center," *Journal of the American Medical Informatics Association,* Vol. 9, No. 5, 2002, pp. 529–539.

Moore, P., "Does Your EMR = ROI? These Systems Can Save You Money, Eventually," *Shands Healthcare Physicians Practice Digest,* 2002.

National Imaging Associates, *NIA's RADMD Portal Uses Web to Improve Efficiency,* Hackensack, N.J., 2000. Available online at http://www.sybase.com/content/1010850/RADMD.pdf (as of February 14, 2005).

Norbut, M., "Healthy Investments," *Commercial Investments Real Estate (CIRE),* 2004.

North Fulton Family Medicine, *Primary Care Davies Award,* 2004. Available online at http://www.himss.org/content/files/davies2004_primarycare_northFulton.pdf (as of May 22, 2005).

Ober, S., *Hearing on the Confidentiality of Patient Records,* Testimony Before the Subcommittee on Health of the House Committee on Ways and Means, Washington, D.C., 2000. Available online at waysandmeans.house.gov/legacy/health/106cong/2-17-00/2-17ober.htm (as of February 14, 2005).

Old Harding Pediatrics Associates, *Primary Care Davies Award,* 2004. Available online at http://www.himss.org/content/files/davies2004_primarycare_oldHarding.pdf (as of May 22, 2005).

Pediatrics @ the Basin, *Primary Care Davies Award,* 2004, online at http://www.himss.org/content/files/davies2004_primarycare_Pediatrics.pdf (as of May 22, 2005).

Phelan, J., "Pay Incentives to Physicians for Filing Electronic Claims," *Managed Care,* Vol. 12, No. 10, 2003, pp. 32–36.

Pifer, E., S. Smith, and G. W. Keever, "EMR to the Rescue," *Healthcare Informatics,* 2001.

Pontius, A., "Talking with Kenneth Freeman of Quest Diagnostics—In the Eyes of the Experts—Medical Laboratory Industry," *Medical Laboratory Observer,* 2002.

Quinn, R., "Transaction Portal Cuts Costs," *Health Management Technology,* 2003.

Riverpoint Pediatrics, *Primary Care Davies Award,* 2004. Available online at http://www.himss.org/content/files/davies2004_primarycare_riverpoint.pdf (as of May 22, 2005).

Roswell Pediatric Center, *Primary Care Davies Award,* 2003. Available online at http://www.himss.org/content/files/davies_2003_primarycare_roswell.pdf (as of May 22, 2005).

Rouse, R., and J. Chalson, *The Evolution of eHealth,* New York: Lehman Brothers, 2000.

Sandrick, K., "Calculating ROI for CPRs," *Health Management Technology,* Vol. 19, No. 6, 1998, pp. 16–20.

SMG Marketing Group, "Chains Dominate DIC Market," *SMG Market Letter,* Vol. 14, No. 10, 2000.

Spetz, J., and R. Given, "The Future of the Nurse Shortage: Will Wage Increases Close the Gap?" *Health Affairs,* Vol. 22, No. 6, 2003, pp. 199–205.

Sunshine, J., M. Mabry, and S. Bansal, "The Volume and Cost of Radiologic Services in the United States in 1990," *American Journal of Roentgenology,* Vol. 157, 1991, pp. 609–613.

Tang, J., V. Grover, and W. Guttler, "Information Technology Innovations: General Diffusion Patterns and Its Relationship to Innovation Characteristics," *IEEE Transactions on Engineering Management,* Vol. 49, No. 1, 2002, pp. 13–27.

Taylor, R., A. Bower, F. Girosi, et al., "Promoting Health Information Technology: Is There a Case for More-Aggressive Government Action," *Health Affairs,* Vol. 24, No. 5, September 14, 2005.

Tierney, W., and M. Miller, "Physician Inpatient Order Writing on Microcomputer Workstations. Effects on Resource Utilization," *JAMA,* Vol. 269, No. 3, 1993, pp. 379–383.

Uehling, M., "Winona, Web Forge Healthy Connection," *College of American Pathologists,* Vol. 15, No. 1, 2001, pp. 58–62.

Verispan/SMG Marketing Group, *Diagnostic Imaging Center Directory,* Chicago, Ill., 2004. Available online at http://www.alphateam.com/medpros.php?md=diagimg (as of February 14, 2005).

Versel, N., "St. Francis Hospital Goes Digital on Time and on Budget," *Health-IT World Newsletter,* 2004. Available online at http://www.health-itworld.com/enews/09-16-2004_405.html (as of May 22, 2005).

Wang, S., et al., "A Cost-Benefit Analysis of Electronic Medical Records in Primary Care," *The American Journal of Medicine,* Vol. 114, 2003, pp. 397–403.

Wiley, G., "Multisite Freestanding Imaging: Is More Better?" *Decisions in Imaging Economics,* 2004. Available online at http://www.imagingeconomics.com/library/200411-04.asp (as of February 14, 2005).

Wong, D., et al., "Changes in Intensive Care Unit Nurse Task Activity After Installation of a Third-Generation Intensive Care Unit Information System," *Critical Care Medicine,* Vol. 31, No. 10, 2003, pp. 2488–2494.

Workgroup for Electronic Data Interchange, *The WEDI Report 1993,* WEDI, 1993. Available online at http://www.wedi.org/public/articles/full1993report.doc (as of February 14, 2005).

Wu, R., W. Peters, and M. Morgan, "The Next Generation of Clinical Decision Support: Linking Evidence to Best Practice," *Journal of Healthcare Information Management,* Vol. 16, No. 4, 2002, pp. 50–55.